Sinusitis

The Complete Guide to Diagnosis and Treatment

Kian M. Hart

Xspurts.com

A New Zealand Designed Product

Other Versions Available

Why limit yourself to just one format?

This book is now available in physical, digital, and audiobook options.

Choose the way you love to read and dive into the story today. You won't regret it!

Digital ISBN: 9781776848010
Physical ISBN: 9781776846924
Audio ISBN:

To obtain a different format of this book at a discounted price, please get in touch with us at:

http://isbn.xspurts.com/

Contents

Have Questions / Comments? 1

Get Free Stuff 3

1. Introduction 5
2. Understanding Sinusitis 8
3. What is Sinusitis? 14
4. Causes and Risk Factors 29
5. Symptoms and Diagnosis 41
6. Over, the, Counter Treatments 50
7. Prescription Treatments 59
8. Home Remedies and Lifestyle Changes 69
9. Surgical Options 81
10. Post, Surgery Care and Recovery 91
11. Prevention Strategies 101
12. Sinusitis in Children 111
13. Sinusitis and Other Health Conditions 121
14. Mental Health and Sinusitis 132
15. The Role of Diet and Nutrition 143
16. Understanding Allergies and Sinusitis 154

17. The Future of Sinusitis Treatment 165

18. Living with Sinusitis 176

19. Resources and Support 187

20. Sinusitis and the Immune System 199

21. The Role of Exercise in Sinus Health 209

22. Complementary and Alternative Treatments 219

23. Sinusitis and the Weather 229

24. Sinusitis and Travel 239

25. Pregnancy and Sinusitis 250

26. The Impact of Pollution on Sinusitis 261

27. Understanding Your Sinusitis Triggers 272

28. Sinusitis Myths and Misconceptions 283

29. Your Sinusitis Action Plan 293

Have Questions / Comments?

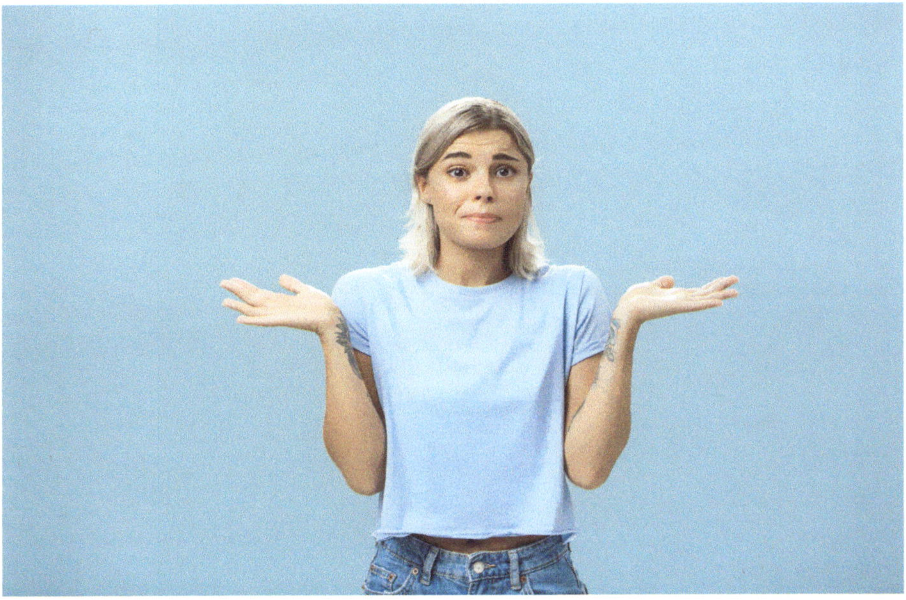

This book was designed to cover as much information as possible, but I know I have probably missed something, or some new amazing discovery has just come out.

If you notice something missing or have a question that I failed to answer, please get in touch and let me know. If I can, I will email you an answer and also update the book so others can also benefit from it.

Thanks For Being Awesome :)

Submit Your Questions / Comments At:

https://questions.xspurts.com

Get Free Stuff

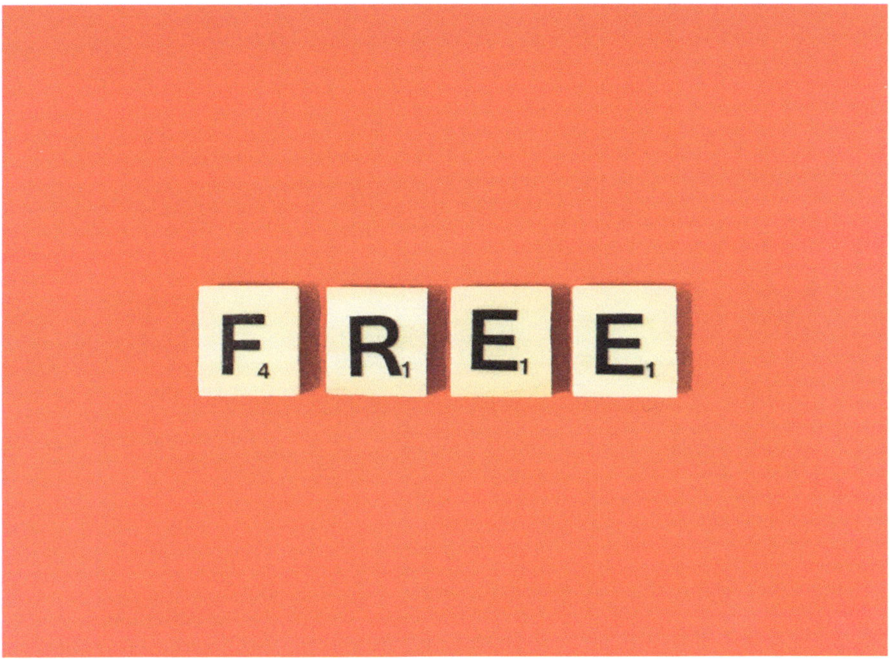

We love writing and have produced a huge number of books.

For being one of our amazing readers, we would love to offer you more books we have created, 100% free.

To claim this limited time special offer, simply go to the site below and enter your name and email address.

You will then receive loads (as we love our readers so much :) of our great books, content and audio direct to your email account, 100% free!

Get Loads of FREE Stuff at:

https://free.xspurts.com

Chapter One

Introduction

Ah, sinusitis. The condition that turns even the most stoic among us into a sniffling, sneezing, congested mess. It's the ultimate party pooper, the unwelcome guest that never seems to leave. But fear not, my friend, because this book is here to help you understand sinusitis with empathy and a healthy dose of humor.

Understanding Sinusitis

Before we can tackle sinusitis, we need to understand what it is and how it affects our bodies. This chapter will explore the anatomy and function of the sinuses, as well asthe types of sinusitis , from acute to chronic, and the common causes and risk factors that can trigger it.

Symptoms and Diagnosis

Ah, the joys of sinusitis symptoms. From headaches to facial pain to that never, ending congestion, we've all been there. This chapter will delve into the most common symptoms, complications, and diagnostic tests that doctors use to diagnose sinusitis.

Treatment Options

When it comes to sinusitis, there are a variety of treatment options, from over, the, counter remedies to prescription medications and even surgical options. This chapter will explore the different treatments available, including home remedies and lifestyle changes, as well as the latest advances in sinus surgery.

Prevention and Management

Prevention is always better than cure, and in this chapter, we'll discuss the best strategies for preventing sinusitis before it even starts. We'll explore the role of diet and nutrition, exercise, and the immune system in sinus health, as well as the importance of good hygiene and avoiding allergens and irritants.

Living with Sinusitis

Sinusitis can be a chronic condition, and managing its symptoms can be a challenge. This chapter will explore the best practices for managing symptoms and staying active while living with sinusitis. We'll also discuss the impact of sinusitis on mental health and the resources and support available for those who need it.

Myths and Misconceptions

From the idea that sinusitis is just a fancy name for a cold to the belief that antibiotics are a cure, all, there are plenty of myths and misconceptions surrounding sinusitis. In this chapter, we'll dispel common myths and provide the truth about sinusitis to help you better manage your condition.

Your Sinusitis Action Plan

In this final chapter, we'll help you develop a personalized management plan for your sinusitis. We'll discuss when to seek medical help, how to identify your triggers, and the best strategies for staying proactive in your sinus health. With the right action plan, you can take control of your sinusitis and get back to feeling like yourself again.

Whether you're a sinusitis veteran or a newcomer to the world of sinus problems, this book is here to provide you with the information, empathy, and humor you need to navigate the challenges of living with sinusitis. So grab a box of tissues and let's dive in!

Chapter Two

Understanding Sinusitis

Sinusitis is a common condition that affects millions of people worldwide. It is characterized by inflammation and swelling of the sinus passages, which can cause a range of symptoms and discomfort. Below we will explore the various aspects of sinusitis, including its causes, symptoms, diagnosis, and treatment options.

The sinuses are hollow cavities located in the facial bones surrounding the nasal area. They are lined with mucous membranes that produce mucus to help moisten and clean the air we breathe. However, when these sinuses become inflamed or infected, it can lead to sinusitis.

There are several factors that can contribute to the development of sinusitis. One of the most common causes is a viral infection, such as the common cold or the flu. Bacterial infections can also cause sinusitis, particularly when they follow a viral infection. Other factors that can increase the risk of sinusitis include allergies, nasal polyps, a deviated septum, and structural abnormalities in the sinuses.

The symptoms of sinusitis can vary from person to person and may include nasal congestion, facial pain or pressure, headache, cough, postnasal drip, and reduced sense of smell. These symptoms can be bothersome and affect a person's quality of life. In some cases, sinusitis can also lead to complications such as chronic sinusitis, sinus infections, and the spread of infection to other parts of the body.

Diagnosing sinusitis typically involves a thorough evaluation of a person's symptoms, medical history, and a physical examination. In some cases, additional tests such as nasal endoscopy, imaging studies (such as CT scans), or allergy tests may be recommended to determine the underlying cause of sinusitis.

Treatment options for sinusitis depend on the underlying cause and severity of the condition. For mild cases, self, care measures such as rest, hydration, saline nasal rinses, and over, the, counter pain relievers can help alleviate symptoms and promote healing. In cases where bacterial infection is suspected, antibiotics may be prescribed. For chronic or recurrent sinusitis, other treatment options such as nasal corticosteroids, antihistamines, and immunotherapy may be recommended. In severe cases or when complications arise, surgery may be necessary to remove obstructions or correct structural abnormalities in the sinuses.

Preventing sinusitis is possible by taking certain precautions. Maintaining good nasal hygiene, such as rinsing the nasal passages with saline solution, can help flush out irritants and promote sinus health. Avoiding known allergens, such as dust mites, pollen, or pet dander, can also reduce the risk of sinusitis in individuals with allergies. Quitting smoking and reducing exposure to environmental irritants can further decrease the likelihood of developing sinusitis.

It's important to note that sinusitis can be a recurring condition for some individuals, requiring ongoing management and prevention strategies. This may include regular follow, up with a healthcare provider, adherence to prescribed medications, and lifestyle modifications to minimize triggers and maintain sinus health.

Anatomy of the Sinuses

The sinuses are fascinating structures within our skull that play a vital role in our overall health. They are a system of interconnected hollow spaces lined with mucous membranes, located in the facial bones surrounding the nasal area. Below we will explore the anatomy of the sinuses and how their structure relates to the development of sinusitis.

There are four pairs of sinuses in the human skull: the frontal sinuses, ethmoid sinuses, sphenoid sinuses, and maxillary sinuses. Each pair of sinuses has its own unique shape, size, and location, but they all serve important functions.

Let's start with the frontal sinuses, which are located in the forehead area, just above the eyes. These sinuses are relatively small and can vary in size among individuals. They are connected to the nasal cavity through small openings called ostia. The frontal sinuses help to lighten the weight of the skull and provide protection to the brain.

Moving to the ethmoid sinuses, they are situated between the eyes and behind the bridge of the nose. The ethmoid sinuses consist of a series of small air cells that are separated by thin bony walls. These sinuses are essential for the production and secretion of mucus, which helps to moisturize the nasal passages and trap dust particles and allergens.

The sphenoid sinuses, as the name suggests, are located within the sphenoid bone at the base of the skull. They are situated behind the ethmoid sinuses and in close proximity to the pituitary gland, a vital endocrine gland. The sphenoid sinuses help to regulate the pressure in the skull and provide resonance to the voice.

Finally, we have the maxillary sinuses, which are the largest of the sinus cavities. They are located in the cheekbones, on either side of the nose. The maxillary sinuses have a pyramidal shape and are responsible for draining mucus into the nasal cavity. They also help to warm and humidify the air we breathe.

The structure of the sinuses is intricately connected to the development of sinusitis. Sinusitis occurs when the sinuses become inflamed and infected, leading to symptoms such as nasal congestion, facial pain, headache, and postnasal drip. Several factors can contribute to the development of sinusitis, including viral or bacterial infections, allergies, structural abnormalities, and environmental irritants.

The interconnectedness of the sinuses is both a blessing and a challenge when it comes to sinusitis. On one hand, the narrow openings that connect the sinuses to the nasal cavity can easily become blocked, preventing proper drainage and leading to the accumulation of mucus and bacteria. This can result in the development of sinus infections. On the other hand, the interconnected nature of the sinuses allows for the spread of infection from one sinus to another.

Understanding the anatomy of the sinuses is crucial in diagnosing and treating sinusitis. Healthcare providers may use imaging techniques such as CT scans to visualize the sinuses and assess their condition. By identifying any structural abnormalities or blockages, they can develop a targeted treatment plan to alleviate symptoms and promote healing.

Function of the Sinuses

The sinuses, those air, filled cavities within our skull, serve various important functions in our bodies. While many people associate the sinuses solely with sinusitis and the discomfort it brings, it's crucial to recognize their broader purpose. Below we will explore the functions of the sinuses and their relation to sinusitis, shedding light on these often, underestimated structures.

The primary function of the sinuses is to produce mucus, a slimy substance that moisturizes and protects the nasal passages. The mucous membranes that line the sinuses secrete mucus to help keep the nasal passages moist, preventing dryness and irritation. This moist environment is essential for maintaining healthy nasal tissues and preventing infections.

Mucus also acts as a filter, trapping dust particles, allergens, and other pollutants present in the air we breathe. By capturing these particles, mucus prevents them from reaching deeper into the respiratory system, thus reducing the risk of respiratory issues and allergic reactions.

Another vital function of the sinuses is to lighten the weight of the skull. The hollow spaces of the sinuses help to reduce the overall weight of the skull while maintaining its structural integrity. This lightening effect contributes to easier head movements and prevents unnecessary strain on the neck and facial muscles.

Furthermore, the sinuses play a role in producing resonance in our voices. As air passes through the sinuses, it resonates and modifies the sound produced by the vocal cords. This adds richness and depth to our voice, influencing our speech patterns and vocal quality.

However, the same characteristics that make the sinuses beneficial can also contribute to the development of sinusitis. Sinusitis occurs when the sinuses become inflamed and infected, leading to symptoms such as nasal congestion, facial pain, pressure, and headaches. Factors such as infections, allergies, anatomical abnormalities, and environmental irritants can disrupt the normal functioning of the sinuses, causing inflammation and a blockage of the sinus openings.

When the sinus openings are blocked, mucus cannot drain properly, leading to its accumulation within the sinuses. This stagnant mucus provides a breeding ground for bacteria, leading to infection and the characteristic symptoms of sinusitis. The inflammation in the sinuses can also cause swelling and increased mucus production, exacerbating the symptoms and further hindering proper sinus drainage.

Understanding the functions of the sinuses is crucial in managing and preventing sinusitis. Maintaining the health of the sinuses involves several key strategies. First, ensuring adequate hydration helps to keep the mucus thin and promotes proper drainage. Drinking plenty of fluids throughout the day can help prevent mucus from becoming thick and sticky, reducing the risk of sinus blockages.

Secondly, managing allergies effectively is essential. Allergies can trigger inflammation in the sinuses and worsen symptoms of sinusitis. Identifying and avoiding allergens, using medications as prescribed by a healthcare provider, and practicing good allergy management techniques can help minimize sinusitis flare, ups.

Additionally, maintaining good nasal hygiene is crucial for sinus health. This includes regularly washing the nasal passages with saline solutions or using a nasal rinse device to flush out irritants, allergens, and excess mucus. These practices help to keep the sinuses clean and reduce the risk of inflammation and infection.

Chapter Three

What is Sinusitis?

Sinusitis is a common condition that affects millions of people worldwide. It refers to the inflammation or swelling of the sinuses, which are the air, filled cavities in the skull connected to the nasal passages. This condition can cause a range of symptoms and discomfort, impacting daily life and overall well, being. Below we will explore the definition, causes, symptoms, and treatment options for sinusitis, shedding light on this prevalent condition.

Sinusitis occurs when the sinuses become inflamed or infected, leading to a blockage of the sinus passages. This blockage prevents proper drainage of mucus, causing it to accumulate within the sinuses. The trapped mucus creates a favorable environment for bacteria, viruses, or fungi to grow, leading to an infection. The condition can be acute, lasting for a short period, or chronic, persisting for several weeks or even months.

There are several factors that can contribute to the development of sinusitis. Common causes include:

Viral or bacterial infections: Sinusitis can be a complication of common colds, flu, or other respiratory infections. The viruses or bacteria can cause inflammation and lead to sinus blockage and infection.

Allergies: Individuals with allergic rhinitis or other allergies are more prone to developing sinusitis. Allergens such as pollen, dust mites, or pet dander can trigger an allergic reaction, leading to sinus inflammation.

Structural abnormalities: Certain structural issues in the nasal passages or sinuses can obstruct proper drainage and increase the risk of sinusitis. Examples include deviated septum, nasal polyps, or narrow sinus openings.

Environmental factors: Exposure to irritants such as pollutants, cigarette smoke, or chemical fumes can irritate the nasal passages and sinuses, leading to inflammation.

The symptoms of sinusitis can vary depending on the duration and severity of the condition. Common symptoms include:

Nasal congestion and stuffiness: The blockage of the sinus passages can cause difficulty in breathing through the nose, leading to a feeling of congestion and stuffiness.

Facial pain or pressure: Sinusitis can cause discomfort or pressure in the face, particularly around the eyes, cheeks, and forehead. This pain may worsen with certain movements or changes in position.

Headache: Many individuals with sinusitis experience headaches, which can range from mild to severe. The pain is often localized around the affected sinuses.

Thick nasal discharge: Sinusitis can cause a thick, discolored nasal discharge that may drain down the throat or cause a post, nasal drip. This discharge may be accompanied by a reduced sense of smell or taste.

Cough: Sinusitis can trigger a persistent cough, particularly at night, as the accumulated mucus irritates the throat.

Fatigue and malaise: The constant discomfort and disrupted sleep due to sinusitis can lead to feelings of fatigue and general malaise.

When it comes to treating sinusitis, the approach depends on the underlying cause and the severity of the symptoms. Mild cases of acute sinusitis often resolve on their own with rest, hydration, and over, the, counter pain relievers. However, if the symptoms persist or worsen, medical intervention may be necessary.

Treatment options for sinusitis include:

Nasal irrigation: Saline nasal irrigation using a neti pot or nasal spray can help flush out mucus and relieve congestion.

Decongestants: Over, the, counter decongestant medications can provide temporary relief by reducing nasal congestion.

Pain relievers: Nonsteroidal anti, inflammatory drugs (NSAIDs) or acetaminophen can help alleviate pain and reduce inflammation.

Types of Sinusitis

Sinusitis is a common condition characterized by inflammation or infection of the sinuses. While most people are familiar with the term "sinusitis," it is important to note that there are different types of sinusitis, each with its own characteristics and treatment approaches. Below we will explore the various types of sinusitis, shedding light on their unique features and considerations.

Acute Sinusitis: This is the most common type of sinusitis and typically lasts for a short duration, usually less than four weeks. It is often caused by a viral infection, such as the common cold or flu. Acute sinusitis can also occur as a result of a bacterial infection. Symptoms include facial pain or pressure, nasal congestion, thick nasal discharge, and a reduced sense of smell. Treatment for acute sinusitis may involve rest, hydration, over, the, counter pain relievers, and nasal irrigation. In some cases, antibiotics may be prescribed if a bacterial infection is present.

Chronic Sinusitis: Chronic sinusitis is diagnosed when the symptoms persist for more than 12 weeks, despite medical treatment. It is often associated with underlying conditions such as allergies, nasal polyps, or structural abnormalities in the nasal passages. The symptoms of chronic sinusitis are similar to acute sinusitis but may be less severe. They include nasal congestion, post, nasal drip, facial pain, and fatigue. Treatment for chronic sinusitis may involve a combination of medications, nasal sprays, saline irrigation, and in some cases, surgery to correct any structural issues.

Subacute Sinusitis: Subacute sinusitis is a condition that falls between acute and chronic sinusitis. It typically lasts for more than four weeks but less than 12 weeks. The symptoms are similar to those of acute sinusitis but may be slightly milder or linger for a longer period. The treatment for subacute sinusitis is similar to that of acute sinusitis and may involve nasal irrigation, decongestants, and pain relievers.

Recurrent Sinusitis: Recurrent sinusitis refers to multiple episodes of acute sinusitis within a year. It is characterized by repeated episodes of sinus inflammation and infection, with periods of symptom, free intervals in between. The underlying causes of recurrent sinusitis may include allergies, anatomical abnormalities, or immune system disorders. Managing recurrent sinusitis involves identifying and addressing the underlying causes, such as allergy management, nasal sprays, and potential surgical interventions.

Fungal Sinusitis: Fungal sinusitis is a less common type of sinusitis caused by a fungal infection. It can occur in individuals with compromised immune systems, such as those with uncontrolled diabetes or HIV/AIDS. Fungal sinusitis may present with chronic symptoms, such as nasal congestion, facial pain, and thick nasal discharge. Treatment often involves antifungal medications and addressing any underlying immune system issues.

Allergic Fungal Sinusitis: Allergic fungal sinusitis is a specific type of fungal sinusitis that occurs in individuals with allergies. It is characterized by a hypersensitivity reaction to fungal spores in the sinuses, leading to chronic inflammation and nasal polyps. Symptoms may include nasal congestion, nasal polyps, reduced sense of smell, and facial pain. Treatment may involve a combination of antifungal medications, allergy management, and possibly surgery to remove nasal polyps.

It is important to note that self, diagnosis of sinusitis is not recommended. If you suspect you have sinusitis or if your symptoms persist or worsen, it is advisable to seek medical attention. A healthcare provider can accurately diagnose the type of sinusitis and recommend appropriate treatment options based on your specific condition.

Acute Sinusitis

Acute Sinusitis: Unmasking the Discomfort

Sinusitis is a prevalent condition that affects millions of individuals worldwide. Among the various types of sinusitis, acute sinusitis stands out as a commonly encountered and disruptive form. Below we will delve into the depths of acute sinusitis, shedding light on its definition, causes, symptoms, and treatment options, as well as its impact on daily life.

Acute sinusitis, also known as acute rhinosinusitis, refers to the sudden onset of inflammation or infection of the sinuses. The sinuses are hollow cavities located in the bones around the nose and eyes. They are lined with mucous membranes that produce mucus to moisten and protect the nasal passages. However, when these sinuses become inflamed or infected, the normal flow of mucus is obstructed, leading to a buildup of mucus and subsequent symptoms.

The most common cause of acute sinusitis is a viral infection, often triggered by the same viruses responsible for the common cold or influenza. These viral infections can cause the nasal passages and sinuses to become swollen and blocked, hindering the proper drainage of mucus. This blockage creates an ideal environment for bacteria to multiply, leading to a secondary bacterial infection in some cases. Less commonly, acute sinusitis can also be caused directly by bacteria or fungal organisms.

The symptoms of acute sinusitis can vary in severity and duration, but typically last for less than four weeks. They may include:

Nasal congestion: A feeling of stuffiness or blockage in the nose, making it difficult to breathe through the nostrils.

Thick nasal discharge: Mucus production increases in response to the infection, resulting in a thick, yellow or greenish discharge from the nose.

Facial pain or pressure: The inflamed sinuses can cause discomfort or pressure in the face, particularly around the eyes, cheeks, and forehead. This pain may worsen with bending forward or lying down.

Loss of smell: The inflammation and congestion can lead to a reduced sense of smell, affecting one's ability to fully appreciate aromas.

Headache: The pressure and inflammation in the sinuses can cause headaches, which may be localized in the forehead, temples, or behind the eyes.

Fatigue: The body's immune response to the infection can lead to a feeling of tiredness or general malaise.

While acute sinusitis can be uncomfortable and disruptive, it is typically a self, limiting condition that resolves on its own without medical intervention. However, there are steps one can take to manage the symptoms and speed up recovery:

Rest: Getting adequate rest allows the body to focus its energy on fighting the infection and healing.

Hydration: Drinking plenty of fluids, such as water or warm herbal teas, helps to thin mucus and promote proper drainage.

Nasal irrigation: Using saline nasal sprays or performing nasal rinses with a neti pot can help flush out mucus and relieve congestion.

Warm compresses: Applying warm compresses to the face can help alleviate facial pain or pressure and promote sinus drainage.

Over, the, counter medications: Nonsteroidal anti, inflammatory drugs (NSAIDs) can help alleviate pain and reduce inflammation. Decongestant nasal sprays or oral decongestants may provide temporary relief from nasal congestion, but should be used sparingly and for short periods to avoid rebound congestion.

In some cases, when symptoms are severe or persistent, medical intervention may be necessary. A healthcare professional may prescribe antibiotics if a bacterial infection is suspected or if symptoms worsen after an initial viral infection. However, it is important to note that antibiotics are not routinely prescribed for uncomplicated acute sinusitis, as the condition is mostly viral.

Subacute Sinusitis

Subacute Sinusitis: Navigating the Middle Ground

When it comes to sinusitis, most people are familiar with acute and chronic forms of the condition. However, there is another category that falls in between: subacute sinusitis. Below we will explore the unique features of subacute sinusitis, including its definition, causes, symptoms, and treatment options.

Subacute sinusitis is characterized by inflammation or infection of the sinuses that persists for more than four weeks but less than 12 weeks. It falls between the relatively short duration of acute sinusitis and the prolonged nature of chronic sinusitis. While the exact cause of subacute sinusitis may vary, it often stems from similar factors as acute sinusitis.

One common cause of subacute sinusitis is a lingering viral infection that does not fully resolve after the acute phase. Viruses such as those responsible for the common cold or influenza can trigger initial sinus inflammation, but the symptoms may persist beyond the typical acute duration. Additionally, subacute sinusitis can occur as a result of bacterial infection or be associated with allergies, nasal polyps, or structural abnormalities in the nasal passages.

The symptoms of subacute sinusitis resemble those of acute sinusitis, but they may be slightly milder or persist for a more extended period. Common symptoms include:

Nasal congestion: A feeling of blockage or stuffiness in the nose, making it difficult to breathe freely.

Thick nasal discharge: Mucus production increases, resulting in a thicker, yellow or greenish discharge from the nose.

Facial pain or pressure: Discomfort or pressure is experienced in the face, often around the cheeks, eyes, and forehead. The pain may worsen with certain movements or changes in position.

Reduced sense of smell: The inflammation and congestion can lead to a diminished sense of smell, affecting the ability to detect odors properly.

Headache: Sinus pressure and inflammation can cause headaches, which may be localized in the forehead or around the eyes.

Fatigue: The body's immune response to the infection and the persistent discomfort can lead to feelings of tiredness or general malaise.

The treatment of subacute sinusitis focuses on alleviating symptoms and addressing any underlying causes. It often involves a combination of self, care measures and medical intervention, depending on the severity and persistence of symptoms. Here are some treatment options that may be recommended:

Nasal irrigation: Regular nasal rinsing with saline solutions or using a neti pot can help flush out mucus and relieve congestion. This practice helps maintain proper sinus drainage and reduce inflammation.

Nasal corticosteroid sprays: Prescription or over, the, counter nasal sprays containing corticosteroids may be recommended to reduce inflammation in the nasal passages and sinuses. These sprays help relieve congestion and improve symptoms.

Decongestants: Short, term use of decongestant nasal sprays or oral decongestants can provide temporary relief by shrinking swollen nasal tissues and reducing congestion. However, they should be used sparingly and for short periods to avoid rebound congestion.

Pain relievers: Nonsteroidal anti, inflammatory drugs (NSAIDs) such as ibuprofen or acetaminophen can help alleviate pain, reduce inflammation, and relieve headaches associated with subacute sinusitis.

Antibiotics: If a bacterial infection is suspected or confirmed, antibiotics may be prescribed. However, they are not routinely prescribed for uncomplicated subacute sinusitis, as most cases are viral in nature.

Allergy management: If allergies are identified as a contributing factor to subacute sinusitis, allergy management techniques such as avoiding triggers, using allergy medications, or undergoing allergen immunotherapy may be recommended.

Chronic Sinusitis

Chronic Sinusitis: A Prolonged Battle with Discomfort

When sinusitis becomes an ongoing struggle, it transitions into a more persistent and challenging form known as chronic sinusitis. Unlike acute sinusitis, which typically lasts for a short period, chronic sinusitis persists for more than 12 weeks, causing significant discomfort and impacting daily life. Below we will explore the intricacies of chronic sinusitis, including its definition, causes, symptoms, and treatment options.

Chronic sinusitis is characterized by inflammation or infection of the sinuses that lasts for an extended period. It is typically caused by underlying factors that hinder the proper functioning of the sinuses, leading to persistent symptoms. These factors may include:

Allergies: Allergic rhinitis or other allergic conditions can trigger chronic inflammation in the nasal passages and sinuses, leading to chronic sinusitis. Allergens such as pollen, dust mites, or pet dander can provoke an immune response and cause ongoing sinus inflammation.

Nasal Polyps: Nasal polyps are small, noncancerous growths that can develop in the lining of the nasal passages and sinuses. They can obstruct the sinus openings, leading to persistent inflammation and impaired sinus drainage.

Structural Abnormalities: Structural issues within the nasal passages or sinuses, such as a deviated septum or narrow sinus openings, can impede proper sinus drainage and contribute to chronic sinusitis.

Respiratory Tract Infections: Recurrent or persistent respiratory tract infections, such as bacterial or fungal infections, can lead to chronic inflammation and sinusitis. These infections may require specific treatments to address the underlying infection.

The symptoms of chronic sinusitis are similar to those of acute sinusitis, but they are often less severe and more persistent. Common symptoms include:

Nasal congestion: A feeling of blockage or stuffiness in the nose that persists for an extended period. This congestion can affect the ability to breathe freely through the nose.

Thick nasal discharge: Persistent production of thick, discolored mucus that drains down the back of the throat or leads to a post, nasal drip.

Facial pain or pressure: Ongoing discomfort or pressure in the face, particularly around the cheeks, eyes, and forehead. This pain may vary in intensity and may be more pronounced in certain positions or during specific activities.

Reduced sense of smell: Chronic inflammation and congestion can result in a diminished sense of smell, affecting the ability to detect odors properly.

Headache: Recurrent headaches, often localized in the forehead or around the eyes, can be a persistent symptom of chronic sinusitis.

Fatigue: The constant inflammation and ongoing symptoms of chronic sinusitis can lead to feelings of tiredness, exhaustion, or general malaise.

The treatment of chronic sinusitis aims to reduce inflammation, promote sinus drainage, and alleviate symptoms. Treatment options may include:

Nasal Corticosteroids: Prescription or over, the, counter nasal sprays containing corticosteroids can help reduce inflammation in the nasal passages and sinuses. These sprays are often used long, term to manage chronic sinusitis and improve symptoms.

Saline Nasal Irrigation: Regular use of saline nasal rinses or nasal irrigation systems helps flush out mucus, reduce inflammation, and promote sinus drainage. This practice can be performed at home and is a vital component of managing chronic sinusitis.

Antibiotics: In cases where a bacterial infection is suspected or confirmed, antibiotics may be prescribed. However, they are not routinely prescribed for uncomplicated chronic sinusitis, as the condition is primarily driven by inflammation rather than infection.

Recurrent Sinusitis

Recurrent Sinusitis: Navigating the Cycle

Sinusitis is a condition that can disrupt daily life and cause discomfort. While acute and chronic sinusitis are well, known forms of the condition, there is another category that affects individuals who experience repeated episodes of sinusitis within a year: recurrent sinusitis. Below we will explore the distinct characteristics of recurrent sinusitis, including its definition, causes, symptoms, and treatment options.

Recurrent sinusitis refers to multiple episodes of acute sinusitis that occur within a 12, month period. It is characterized by recurrent inflammation or infection of the sinuses, leading to the reappearance of symptoms. Individuals with recurrent sinusitis experience periods of symptom, free intervals followed by recurrent flare, ups, causing significant disruptions in their daily lives.

Several factors contribute to the development of recurrent sinusitis:

Allergies: Allergic rhinitis, commonly known as hay fever, is a common trigger for recurrent sinusitis. Exposure to allergens such as pollen, dust mites, or pet dander can cause inflammation in the nasal passages and sinuses, leading to repeated episodes of sinusitis.

Anatomical Abnormalities: Structural abnormalities in the nasal passages or sinuses can obstruct proper sinus drainage and contribute to recurrent sinusitis. Deviated septum, nasal polyps, or narrow sinus openings are examples of such abnormalities that can increase the risk of recurrent episodes.

Nasal Infections: Recurrent viral or bacterial respiratory infections, such as the common cold or flu, can lead to recurrent sinusitis. These infections can trigger inflammation in the sinuses and contribute to repeated episodes.

Environmental Factors: Exposure to environmental irritants such as pollutants, cigarette smoke, or chemical fumes can irritate the nasal passages and sinuses, increasing the likelihood of recurrent sinusitis.

The symptoms of recurrent sinusitis are similar to those of acute sinusitis, but they occur repeatedly over time. Common symptoms include:

Nasal congestion: Persistent or intermittent nasal congestion, making it difficult to breathe through the nose.

Thick nasal discharge: Recurrent production of thick, discolored mucus that may drain down the back of the throat or cause a post, nasal drip.

Facial pain or pressure: Repeated episodes of facial pain or pressure, often centered around the cheeks, eyes, and forehead.

Reduced sense of smell: A diminished sense of smell that recurs with each episode of sinusitis.

Headache: Recurrent headaches, typically localized in the forehead or around the eyes.

Fatigue: Ongoing fatigue and tiredness due to the persistent inflammation and recurrent symptoms.

Managing recurrent sinusitis involves a multifaceted approach tailored to the individual's specific triggers and underlying causes. Treatment options may include:

Allergy Management: If allergies contribute to recurrent sinusitis, identifying and avoiding allergens can help minimize episodes. Allergy medications, such as antihistamines or nasal corticosteroids, may be prescribed to manage allergic symptoms effectively.

Nasal Irrigation: Regular use of saline nasal rinses or nasal irrigation devices helps flush out mucus, reduce inflammation, and promote sinus drainage. This practice can be performed at home and aids in preventing recurrent episodes.

Nasal Corticosteroids: Prescription nasal sprays containing corticosteroids can help reduce inflammation in the nasal passages and sinuses. These sprays are often used long, term to manage chronic inflammation and minimize the frequency of recurrent sinusitis.

Antibiotics: In cases where a bacterial infection is suspected or confirmed, antibiotics may be prescribed to treat the underlying infection. However, antibiotics are not routinely prescribed for uncomplicated recurrent sinusitis.

Chapter Four

Causes and Risk Factors

Causes and Risk Factors: Unmasking the Culprits Behind Sinusitis

Sinusitis is a common condition that affects millions of individuals worldwide. It occurs when the sinuses, the air, filled cavities in the skull, become inflamed or infected. While sinusitis can result from various factors, it is essential to understand the causes and risk factors associated with this condition. Below we will delve into the diverse causes and risk factors of sinusitis, shedding light on the culprits that contribute to its development.

Infections: Infections, particularly viral and bacterial, are among the primary causes of sinusitis. The most common viral infections associated with sinusitis include the common cold and influenza. These infections can lead to inflammation and swelling of the sinuses, hindering proper drainage and creating an ideal environment for bacterial growth. Bacterial sinusitis often occurs as a secondary infection following a viral upper respiratory infection, when the sinuses become vulnerable to bacterial invasion.

Allergies: Allergic rhinitis, commonly known as hay fever, is a significant risk factor for sinusitis. Allergies trigger an immune response in the nasal passages, leading to inflammation and swelling. This inflammation can obstruct the sinus openings, impeding proper drainage and increasing the likelihood of sinusitis. Common allergens include pollen, dust mites, pet dander, and certain foods.

Nasal Abnormalities: Structural abnormalities within the nasal passages and sinuses can contribute to sinusitis. Deviated septum, a condition in which the nasal septum is crooked or off, center, can obstruct sinus drainage and increase the risk of sinusitis. Other anatomical irregularities, such as nasal polyps, tumors, or narrow sinus openings, can also impede proper sinus drainage and airflow, creating an environment conducive to sinusitis.

Respiratory Conditions: Chronic respiratory conditions, such as asthma or chronic obstructive pulmonary disease (COPD), can increase the likelihood of developing sinusitis. These conditions often involve persistent inflammation in the airways, which can extend to the sinuses and lead to chronic sinusitis.

Weakened Immune System: A compromised immune system makes individuals more susceptible to infections, including sinusitis. Conditions that weaken the immune system, such as HIV/AIDS, autoimmune diseases, or immunodeficiency disorders, increase the risk of developing recurrent or chronic sinusitis.

Environmental Irritants: Exposure to environmental irritants can irritate the nasal passages and sinuses, leading to inflammation and increased susceptibility to sinusitis. Irritants include air pollution, cigarette smoke, chemical fumes, and other airborne irritants. Occupational exposure to certain substances, such as wood dust or industrial pollutants, can also contribute to sinusitis.

Dental Infections: Infections in the teeth, particularly in the upper molars, can spread to the adjacent sinuses, leading to sinusitis. These infections can occur as a result of tooth decay, dental abscesses, or gum disease. Proper dental hygiene and prompt treatment of dental infections are essential to prevent sinusitis.

Swimming and Diving: Engaging in activities that involve frequent immersion in water, such as swimming or diving, can increase the risk of sinusitis. Prolonged exposure to water can disrupt the delicate balance of mucus in the sinuses and promote bacterial growth. This is commonly referred to as "swimmer's sinusitis."

It is important to note that while these factors increase the risk of developing sinusitis, they do not guarantee its occurrence. Additionally, the severity and frequency of sinusitis can vary among individuals depending on their susceptibility and exposure to these risk factors.

Understanding the causes and risk factors of sinusitis is crucial in managing and preventing the condition.

Common Cold

The Common Cold: Unveiling the Sneaky Invader

The common cold, often regarded as a minor nuisance, is a prevalent viral infection that affects millions of individuals worldwide. While it is typically seen as a temporary inconvenience, it can sometimes lead to complications such as sinusitis. Below we will explore the common cold in all its sneaky glory, including its definition, causes, symptoms, and its potential connection to sinusitis.

The common cold is an upper respiratory tract infection caused by different strains of viruses, primarily rhinoviruses. These viruses are highly contagious and can be transmitted through respiratory droplets from an infected person, direct contact with contaminated surfaces, or by inhaling airborne particles. The virus enters the body through the nose, mouth, or eyes, where it attaches to the mucous membranes and begins to multiply.

The symptoms of the common cold typically manifest within one to three days after exposure to the virus. They vary from person to person but generally include:

Nasal congestion: The common cold often causes nasal congestion, making it difficult to breathe freely through the nose. This occurs as a result of the inflammation and swelling of the nasal passages.

Runny nose: A runny nose is a common symptom of the common cold. The virus stimulates the production of excess mucus, leading to a watery discharge from the nose.

Sneezing: Sneezing is the body's reflexive response to clear the nasal passages of irritants. It is a common symptom of the common cold and is often triggered by the presence of the virus in the nasal passages.

Sore throat: The viral infection can cause inflammation and irritation of the throat, resulting in a sore or scratchy throat.

Cough: A dry or productive cough may develop as a result of post, nasal drip, where excess mucus from the nasal passages drips down the throat and triggers coughing.

Fatigue and malaise: The immune response to the viral infection can lead to feelings of fatigue, tiredness, and overall malaise.

Now, let's explore the potential connection between the common cold and sinusitis. The common cold can sometimes progress to sinusitis, particularly if there are additional factors at play. Here's how it happens:

When the common cold virus infects the upper respiratory tract, it can cause inflammation and swelling of the nasal passages and sinuses. This inflammation can obstruct the normal flow of mucus, preventing proper sinus drainage. As a result, mucus accumulates in the sinuses, creating an environment conducive to bacterial growth. If the bacterial load becomes significant, it can lead to a secondary bacterial infection, resulting in sinusitis.

However, it is important to note that not every common cold leads to sinusitis. Factors such as individual susceptibility, the virulence of the virus, and the presence of other risk factors play a role in determining whether a cold progresses to sinusitis. For example, individuals with underlying nasal abnormalities, allergies, or weakened immune systems may be more prone to developing sinusitis as a complication of the common cold.

Preventing sinusitis during a common cold involves taking proactive measures to promote proper sinus drainage and minimize bacterial growth. Here are some strategies:

Stay hydrated: Drinking plenty of fluids helps to thin mucus, making it easier to drain from the sinuses. Hydration also supports overall immune function, which can help the body fight off secondary bacterial infections.

Nasal saline rinses: Using saline nasal sprays or performing nasal irrigation with a neti pot can help flush out excess mucus and irritants from the nasal passages, reducing the risk of sinusitis.

Rest and self, care: Taking adequate rest and practicing good self, care, such as getting enough sleep.

Allergic Rhinitis

Allergic Rhinitis: When Allergies Take Center Stage

Allergic rhinitis, also known as hay fever, is a common condition that affects a significant number of individuals worldwide. While it may seem like a mere inconvenience, allergic rhinitis can have a profound impact on one's quality of life and may even lead to complications such as sinusitis. Below we will unravel the intriguing world of allergic rhinitis, exploring its definition, causes, symptoms, and its connection to sinusitis.

Allergic rhinitis is an inflammatory condition of the nasal passages triggered by an immune response to allergens. Allergens are substances that are harmless to most individuals but can provoke an allergic reaction in susceptible individuals. Common allergens include pollen, dust mites, pet dander, mold spores, and certain foods.

The immune response in allergic rhinitis involves the release of histamine and other chemicals, causing inflammation in the nasal passages. This inflammation leads to a range of symptoms that can significantly impact daily life.

The symptoms of allergic rhinitis typically include:

Sneezing: Sneezing is a characteristic symptom of allergic rhinitis. It is a reflexive response aimed at expelling irritants from the nasal passages.

Runny or congested nose: Allergic rhinitis often causes a runny nose, with clear nasal discharge known as rhinorrhea. In some cases, nasal congestion may occur, making it difficult to breathe through the nose.

Itchy nose, throat, or eyes: Individuals with allergic rhinitis often experience itching in the nose, throat, or eyes. This itching sensation can be quite bothersome.

Watery eyes: Allergic rhinitis can lead to increased tear production, resulting in watery or itchy eyes.

Post, nasal drip: Excess mucus produced in the nasal passages may drip down the back of the throat, leading to a sensation of mucus in the throat and causing cough or throat clearing.

Sinus pressure or headache: In some cases, allergic rhinitis can cause sinus pressure or headaches due to the inflammation and congestion in the nasal and sinus cavities.

The connection between allergic rhinitis and sinusitis is noteworthy. When individuals with allergic rhinitis are exposed to allergens, the resulting inflammation and congestion in the nasal passages can obstruct proper sinus drainage. This impaired drainage creates an environment conducive to the development of sinusitis. It is essential to manage allergic rhinitis effectively to minimize the risk of sinusitis.

Here are some strategies for managing allergic rhinitis and reducing the likelihood of sinusitis:

Allergen avoidance: Identifying and avoiding allergens that trigger allergic rhinitis is crucial. For example, individuals with pollen allergies may need to limit outdoor activities during peak pollen seasons, keep windows closed, and use air purifiers to reduce pollen exposure.

Medications: Over, the, counter antihistamines can help alleviate the symptoms of allergic rhinitis by blocking the effects of histamine. Nasal corticosteroid sprays can reduce inflammation and congestion in the nasal passages. Other medications, such as decongestants or leukotriene inhibitors, may be prescribed in certain cases.

Immunotherapy: For individuals with severe allergic rhinitis or inadequate response to medications, allergen immunotherapy (commonly known as allergy shots) may be recommended. This treatment involves gradually exposing the individual to increasing amounts of the allergen, desensitizing the immune system over time.

Nasal irrigation: Regular nasal rinses with saline solutions can help flush out allergens and irritants from the nasal passages, reducing inflammation and promoting proper sinus drainage.

Nasal Polyps

Nasal Polyps: Unraveling the Enigmatic Growth

Nasal polyps are abnormal, noncancerous growths that develop in the lining of the nasal passages or sinuses. While they may sound mysterious, they are a common condition that affects a significant number of individuals. Nasal polyps can have a profound impact on one's quality of life, often leading to complications such as sinusitis. Below we will delve into the intriguing world of nasal polyps, exploring their definition, causes, symptoms, and their connection to sinusitis.

Nasal polyps are soft, painless growths that develop as a result of chronic inflammation in the nasal passages or sinuses. They typically occur in the area where the sinuses and nasal passages meet. Although their exact cause is not fully understood, nasal polyps are often associated with certain conditions and risk factors.

Chronic inflammation plays a crucial role in the development of nasal polyps. The inflammation can be triggered by various factors, including:

Chronic Sinusitis: Nasal polyps are commonly found in individuals with chronic sinusitis, a condition characterized by persistent inflammation of the sinuses. The chronic inflammation leads to swelling and thickening of the sinus lining, creating an environment conducive to the development of polyps.

Allergic Rhinitis: Individuals with allergic rhinitis, commonly known as hay fever, have a higher risk of developing nasal polyps. The chronic inflammation in the nasal passages caused by allergic reactions can contribute to polyp formation.

Asthma: There is a strong association between nasal polyps and asthma. Chronic inflammation in the airways, characteristic of asthma, can extend to the nasal passages and sinuses, increasing the likelihood of nasal polyp development.

In addition to these underlying conditions, several risk factors are associated with an increased likelihood of nasal polyp formation:

Age and Gender: Nasal polyps can occur at any age, but they are more commonly seen in adults, particularly those over the age of 40. Men are more prone to developing nasal polyps than women.

Genetics: There is evidence to suggest that genetic factors play a role in the development of nasal polyps. Individuals with a family history of nasal polyps or certain inflammatory conditions may have a higher predisposition to develop them.

Aspirin Sensitivity: Some individuals with nasal polyps may experience a sensitivity or intolerance to aspirin and other nonsteroidal anti, inflammatory drugs (NSAIDs). This condition, known as aspirin, exacerbated respiratory disease (AERD) or Samter's triad, is characterized by nasal polyps, asthma, and sensitivity to aspirin and NSAIDs.

The symptoms of nasal polyps can vary in severity, and some individuals may not experience any symptoms at all. However, when symptoms do occur, they can significantly impact one's daily life. Common symptoms of nasal polyps include:

Nasal congestion: Nasal polyps can obstruct the nasal passages, leading to chronic nasal congestion or a blocked sensation. Breathing through the nose becomes difficult, and the voice may develop a nasal quality.

Runny nose: Excess mucus production is a common symptom of nasal polyps, leading to a persistent runny nose with thin, watery discharge.

Reduced sense of smell: Nasal polyps can interfere with the sense of smell, causing a partial or complete loss of the ability to detect odors.

Post, nasal drip: Excess mucus produced by the nasal polyps may drip down the back of the throat, leading to a sensation of mucus in the throat and causing coughing or throat clearing.

Deviated Septum

Deviated Septum: When the Nose Takes a Crooked Path

The nose is a remarkable organ that serves multiple functions, including breathing, smelling, and filtering the air we inhale. However, sometimes the structure of the nose is not perfectly aligned, leading to a condition known as a deviated septum. A deviated septum occurs when the thin wall between the nostrils, called the nasal septum, is crooked or displaced. This seemingly minor abnormality can have a significant impact on nasal function and may contribute to complications such as sinusitis. Below we will explore the intriguing world of the deviated septum, including its definition, causes, symptoms, and its connection to sinusitis.

A deviated septum can be congenital, meaning it is present at birth, or it can result from nasal trauma or injury. The nasal septum is made up of cartilage and bone, and if it develops an irregular shape, it can cause the septum to deviate to one side, obstructing the nasal passages to varying degrees. While some individuals have a mild deviation that doesn't cause significant problems, others may experience more pronounced symptoms.

The primary cause of a deviated septum is nasal trauma or injury. It can result from accidents, contact sports, falls, or any forceful impact to the nose. Trauma can cause the nasal septum to become misaligned or crooked, affecting the normal airflow through the nose. In some cases, a deviated septum may be present from birth due to factors such as fetal development or genetic predisposition.

The symptoms of a deviated septum can vary depending on the severity of the deviation. Common symptoms include:

Nasal congestion: A deviated septum can obstruct one or both sides of the nasal passages, leading to chronic nasal congestion. This congestion can make it difficult to breathe through the nose and may result in mouth breathing.

Difficulty breathing: The obstruction caused by a deviated septum can make it challenging to get enough air through the nose. This can lead to a sensation of breathlessness, especially during physical exertion or at night when lying down.

Recurrent sinus infections: The obstruction and impaired airflow caused by a deviated septum can contribute to the development of sinusitis. When the sinuses cannot properly drain, mucus can build up, leading to recurrent infections, facial pain, and pressure.

Nosebleeds: Individuals with a deviated septum may be more prone to nosebleeds due to the disruption of the delicate blood vessels in the nasal septum.

Snoring: A deviated septum can disrupt normal airflow, leading to turbulent airflow during sleep and resulting in snoring.

Sleep apnea: In some cases, a deviated septum can contribute to sleep apnea, a sleep disorder characterized by pauses in breathing during sleep. The obstruction in the nasal passages can make it harder to maintain a clear airway, leading to breathing difficulties during sleep.

It is important to note that not everyone with a deviated septum experiences symptoms. In fact, it is estimated that a significant portion of the population has some degree of septal deviation without being aware of it.

The connection between a deviated septum and sinusitis is noteworthy. The obstruction caused by a deviated septum can interfere with proper sinus drainage. When mucus cannot efficiently exit the sinuses, it can become stagnant, leading to a higher risk of sinusitis. The stagnant mucus creates an ideal environment for bacterial growth and can contribute to recurrent or chronic sinus infections.

Treatment options for a deviated septum depend on the severity of symptoms and the impact on daily life. In mild cases where symptoms are tolerable, conservative measures may be recommended.

Chapter Five

Symptoms and Diagnosis

Symptoms and Diagnosis of Sinusitis: Decoding the Signs of Nasal Distress

Sinusitis, also known as a sinus infection, is a common condition that affects many individuals at some point in their lives. It occurs when the sinuses, the hollow cavities around the nose, become inflamed or infected. Recognizing the symptoms of sinusitis is crucial for timely diagnosis and appropriate treatment. Below we will delve into the intriguing world of sinusitis symptoms and the diagnostic process, shedding light on the signs of nasal distress.

The symptoms of sinusitis can vary depending on the type and severity of the condition. They can manifest in the following ways:

Nasal congestion: One of the hallmark symptoms of sinusitis is nasal congestion, also known as a stuffy or blocked nose. The inflammation in the sinuses causes swelling of the nasal passages, making it difficult to breathe through the nose.

Sinus pressure or pain: Many individuals with sinusitis experience facial pressure or pain. This discomfort is often localized around the forehead, cheeks, and eyes. The pain may worsen when bending forward or lying down.

Thick nasal discharge: Sinusitis is characterized by the production of thick, discolored nasal discharge. The mucus may be yellow, green, or brown in color, indicating an underlying infection.

Post, nasal drip: Sinusitis can cause excessive mucus production, leading to post, nasal drip. This is when mucus drips down the throat from the back of the nose, causing throat irritation, coughing, or a sore throat.

Reduced sense of smell and taste: The inflammation and congestion in the nasal passages can affect the sense of smell (olfaction) and taste. Many individuals with sinusitis report a diminished ability to detect odors and a reduced perception of taste.

Headache: Sinus headaches are common in individuals with sinusitis. These headaches are typically felt as a deep, dull pain in the forehead, cheeks, or around the eyes. The pain may worsen with movement or changes in atmospheric pressure.

Tooth pain: The proximity of the sinuses to the upper teeth can cause referred pain. Inflammation or infection in the sinuses can lead to toothache, often affecting the upper molars.

It is important to note that these symptoms are not exclusive to sinusitis and can also occur in other conditions, such as the common cold or allergies. However, the persistence and severity of symptoms, along with other factors, can help differentiate sinusitis from other nasal disorders.

Diagnosing sinusitis involves a combination of evaluating symptoms, conducting a physical examination, and, in some cases, using additional diagnostic tools. Here are the main steps in the diagnostic process:

Medical history: The healthcare provider will start by taking a detailed medical history, including information about the nature and duration of symptoms. They may ask about previous episodes of sinusitis, allergies, recent respiratory infections, and exposure to irritants.

Physical examination: A thorough physical examination will be performed, focusing on the nasal passages, sinuses, and associated areas. The healthcare provider may inspect the nasal passages using a nasal speculum or an endoscope. They will look for signs of inflammation, nasal polyps, or structural abnormalities.

Symptom evaluation: The duration and pattern of symptoms are crucial in differentiating acute, subacute, or chronic sinusitis. The healthcare provider will assess the severity and frequency of symptoms, including nasal congestion, nasal discharge, facial pain or pressure, and associated symptoms like headache or cough.

Imaging studies: In certain cases, imaging studies may be recommended to visualize the sinuses in more detail.

Common Symptoms

Common Symptoms of Sinusitis: Decoding the Distress within the Sinuses

Sinusitis, a condition characterized by inflammation or infection of the sinuses, can cause a range of distressing symptoms. The sinuses are air, filled cavities located in the facial bones surrounding the nose and eyes. When they become inflamed or infected, they can lead to various symptoms that can significantly impact daily life. Below we will unravel the intriguing world of sinusitis symptoms, shedding light on the common signs of sinus distress.

Nasal Congestion: Nasal congestion, or a stuffy nose, is one of the most common symptoms of sinusitis. The inflammation and swelling of the sinus tissues can cause blockage in the nasal passages, making it difficult to breathe through the nose. This congestion can also contribute to a sensation of pressure or fullness in the face.

Thick Nasal Discharge: Sinusitis often leads to the production of thick, discolored nasal discharge. The mucus may be yellow, green, or brown in color, indicating the presence of an infection. This discharge may drain down the back of the throat, causing a post, nasal drip and associated symptoms such as coughing or a sore throat.

Facial Pain and Pressure: Sinusitis can cause facial pain or pressure, particularly in the areas over the affected sinuses. The pain may be localized around the forehead, cheeks, or between the eyes. The pressure sensation can worsen when bending forward or lying down, as gravity affects the sinus drainage.

Headache: Sinus headaches are a common symptom of sinusitis. The pain is typically felt as a deep, dull ache in the forehead, cheeks, or around the eyes. The headache may worsen with sudden head movements or changes in atmospheric pressure.

Reduced Sense of Smell and Taste: Inflammation and congestion in the nasal passages can affect the sense of smell (olfaction) and taste. Many individuals with sinusitis report a diminished ability to detect odors and a reduced perception of taste. This can impact one's enjoyment of food and beverages.

Toothache: The proximity of the upper teeth to the sinuses can result in referred pain. Sinusitis can cause aching or sensitivity in the upper teeth, often affecting the molars. This pain can be mistaken for a dental issue, leading to unnecessary dental interventions.

Fatigue and Malaise: Sinusitis can leave individuals feeling tired, fatigued, and generally unwell. The body's immune response to infection and the ongoing inflammation can contribute to feelings of fatigue and malaise.

Cough: Sinusitis can trigger a persistent cough, particularly when post, nasal drip occurs. The excess mucus produced in the sinuses may drip down the back of the throat, causing irritation and coughing.

Ear Pressure and Fullness: The close proximity of the sinuses to the ears can result in ear, related symptoms. Sinusitis can cause a sensation of pressure, fullness, or even mild hearing loss in the affected ear(s). This can be due to the congestion and inflammation affecting the Eustachian tubes, which connect the middle ear to the back of the throat.

Bad Breath (Halitosis): Chronic sinusitis can contribute to the development of bad breath, also known as halitosis. The stagnant mucus and the presence of bacteria in the sinuses can lead to an unpleasant odor.

It is important to note that these symptoms can vary in severity and duration, depending on the type and extent of sinusitis. Acute sinusitis typically lasts for a short period (less than 4 weeks), while subacute sinusitis lasts between 4 to 12 weeks.

Complications

Complications of Sinusitis: Unmasking the Hidden Dangers

Sinusitis, a condition characterized by inflammation or infection of the sinuses, can lead to a range of complications that extend beyond the typical symptoms. While most cases of sinusitis resolve with appropriate treatment, certain factors can increase the risk of complications. Below we will explore the intriguing world of sinusitis complications, shedding light on the hidden dangers that can arise.

Acute Bacterial Sinusitis: Acute sinusitis, if left untreated or inadequately managed, can progress to acute bacterial sinusitis. In this condition, the initial viral infection is followed by a secondary bacterial infection. Bacteria invade the sinuses, causing severe symptoms and often requiring more aggressive treatment with antibiotics.

Chronic Sinusitis: When sinusitis persists for 12 weeks or longer, it is classified as chronic sinusitis. This condition can significantly impact an individual's quality of life, leading to persistent symptoms such as nasal congestion, facial pain or pressure, and reduced sense of smell. Chronic sinusitis can be challenging to treat and may require a combination of medications, nasal sprays, and even surgery in severe cases.

Sinusitis and Asthma: Sinusitis and asthma often coexist, and one condition can worsen the other. Chronic sinusitis can trigger or exacerbate asthma symptoms, leading to increased respiratory distress, coughing, and wheezing. The inflammation and mucus production associated with sinusitis can contribute to airway obstruction and difficulty breathing in individuals with asthma.

Sinusitis and Allergies: Individuals with allergic rhinitis or other allergic conditions are more susceptible to sinusitis. The combination of ongoing allergies and sinus inflammation can create a cycle of recurring sinusitis episodes. Allergic reactions can further worsen sinus inflammation, leading to chronic or recurrent sinusitis.

Orbital Cellulitis: Orbital cellulitis is a severe complication of sinusitis that occurs when the infection spreads to the tissues surrounding the eye. The infection can cause eye redness, swelling, pain, and vision changes. Orbital cellulitis is a medical emergency and requires immediate treatment with antibiotics and sometimes surgical drainage.

Osteomyelitis: Osteomyelitis is a rare but serious complication of sinusitis. It occurs when the infection spreads to the bones of the skull, leading to bone inflammation and destruction. Osteomyelitis can cause severe pain, fever, and even neurological symptoms. Prompt treatment with intravenous antibiotics and, in some cases, surgery is necessary to manage this condition.

Meningitis: In rare cases, the infection from sinusitis can spread to the protective membranes covering the brain and spinal cord, leading to meningitis. Meningitis is a life, threatening condition characterized by severe headache, fever, neck stiffness, and neurological symptoms. Immediate medical attention is required for diagnosis and treatment.

Abscess Formation: In some instances, a pus, filled pocket (abscess) can develop within the sinuses. Sinus abscesses can cause severe pain, fever, facial swelling, and even complications like vision changes or neurological symptoms. Drainage of the abscess, along with appropriate antibiotic therapy, is necessary to treat this condition.

Spread of Infection: Sinusitis can lead to the spread of infection to nearby structures, such as the bones of the face, the eye sockets, or the brain. These infections can result in serious complications, including bone infections (osteomyelitis), eye infections (orbital cellulitis), or brain infections (meningitis).

Diagnostic Tests

Diagnostic Tests for Sinusitis: Unveiling the Tools of Detection

Sinusitis, a condition characterized by inflammation or infection of the sinuses, can cause a range of distressing symptoms. To accurately diagnose sinusitis and determine the most appropriate treatment, healthcare providers often rely on various diagnostic tests. These tests help uncover the underlying cause, assess the severity, and guide the management of sinusitis. Below we will delve into the intriguing world of diagnostic tests for sinusitis, shedding light on the tools used to detect and evaluate this common condition.

Medical History and Physical Examination: The diagnostic process for sinusitis typically begins with a comprehensive medical history and physical examination. The healthcare provider will ask detailed questions about symptoms, their duration, and any previous episodes of sinusitis. They will also perform a physical examination, paying particular attention to the nasal passages and facial areas affected by sinusitis. This initial assessment provides valuable clues and helps guide further diagnostic investigations.

Nasal Endoscopy: Nasal endoscopy is a procedure that allows visualization of the nasal passages and sinuses using a thin, flexible tube with a light and camera attached (nasal endoscope). The healthcare provider inserts the endoscope into the nose to examine the nasal cavities, sinus openings, and areas of inflammation or polyp formation. Nasal endoscopy provides a detailed view of the sinuses and can help identify abnormalities, such as nasal polyps or signs of chronic inflammation.

Imaging Studies:

a. X, rays: X, rays were traditionally used to evaluate the sinuses. However, they are now less commonly used due to their limited ability to provide detailed information about the sinuses' internal structures. X, rays can still be helpful in certain cases, particularly when evaluating complications of sinusitis, such as the spread of infection to nearby structures.

b. Computed Tomography (CT) Scan: CT scans are considered the gold standard imaging modality for diagnosing sinusitis. CT scans provide detailed cross, sectional images of the sinuses, allowing healthcare providers to assess the sinuses' size, shape, and any abnormalities, such as mucosal thickening or sinus blockages. CT scans are particularly useful in diagnosing chronic sinusitis, evaluating the extent of disease, and guiding surgical interventions if needed.

c. Magnetic Resonance Imaging (MRI): MRI scans may be used in certain cases to provide detailed images of the sinuses, particularly when assessing complications or suspected structural abnormalities. MRI scans use magnetic fields and radio waves to create detailed images of soft tissues, providing valuable information about the sinuses and surrounding structures.

Nasal Swab Culture: In some cases, a healthcare provider may perform a nasal swab culture to identify the specific bacteria or fungi causing the sinusitis. This involves taking a swab from the nasal passages or sinus cavities and sending it to a laboratory for analysis. Culturing the sample helps identify the causative organism and determine its antibiotic sensitivity, guiding the selection of appropriate antibiotic therapy.

Allergy Testing: Allergy testing may be recommended in individuals with suspected allergic sinusitis or recurring sinusitis triggered by allergens. Allergy tests can help identify specific allergens that may be contributing to sinus inflammation and guide targeted allergen avoidance or immunotherapy.

Blood Tests: Blood tests are not routinely performed for diagnosing sinusitis but may be helpful in certain situations. For example, blood tests can be used to evaluate the body's immune response, detect elevated levels of inflammatory markers, or rule out underlying conditions that may contribute to sinusitis, such as autoimmune disorders or systemic infections.

Nasal Cytology: Nasal cytology involves taking a sample of the nasal discharge or nasal tissue for microscopic examination.

Chapter Six

Over, the, Counter Treatments

Over, the, Counter Treatments for Sinusitis: Empowering Relief at Your Fingertips

Sinusitis, a condition characterized by inflammation or infection of the sinuses, can cause a range of distressing symptoms. While medical intervention is sometimes necessary, many individuals find relief through over, the, counter (OTC) treatments. These accessible and convenient options can help alleviate symptoms and support the body's natural healing process. Below we will delve into the intriguing world of OTC treatments for sinusitis, shedding light on the tools available to empower individuals in their journey toward relief.

Nasal Saline Irrigation: Nasal saline irrigation, often referred to as nasal rinsing or nasal douching, is a simple and effective method for clearing the nasal passages and reducing congestion. It involves flushing the nasal cavities with a saline solution using a squeeze bottle, neti pot, or nasal spray. Saline irrigation helps remove mucus, allergens, and irritants from the sinuses, promoting sinus drainage and reducing inflammation. It can be performed using OTC saline solutions or by making a homemade saline solution with salt and water.

Nasal Decongestant Sprays: Nasal decongestant sprays provide temporary relief from nasal congestion by constricting the blood vessels in the nasal passages. These sprays help reduce swelling and promote better airflow through the nose. However, they should be used with caution and for short periods only, as prolonged use can lead to a rebound effect and worsen congestion. It is important to follow the instructions and not exceed the recommended usage duration.

Nasal Corticosteroid Sprays: Nasal corticosteroid sprays are OTC medications that reduce inflammation in the nasal passages. They work by suppressing the immune response and reducing the swelling of the sinus tissues. Nasal corticosteroid sprays are effective in relieving symptoms such as nasal congestion, runny nose, and sneezing. It is important to use them consistently and as directed to achieve optimal results. These sprays may take a few days to provide noticeable relief, so patience is key.

Oral Decongestants: Oral decongestants are available in pill or liquid form and can provide temporary relief from nasal congestion. These medications work by constricting the blood vessels throughout the body, including those in the nasal passages. They are generally safe for short, term use but should be avoided or used with caution in individuals with certain medical conditions such as high blood pressure or heart problems. It is essential to read and follow the instructions and consult a healthcare professional if necessary.

Pain Relievers: Sinusitis can cause facial pain, pressure, and headaches. OTC pain relievers such as acetaminophen or nonsteroidal anti, inflammatory drugs (NSAIDs) like ibuprofen can help alleviate these symptoms. Pain relievers can also help reduce fever if present. It is important to use these medications according to the recommended dosage and duration, and to consult a healthcare professional if symptoms persist or worsen.

Antihistamines: Antihistamines are commonly used to manage allergic rhinitis symptoms, but they can also provide relief for certain types of sinusitis. They work by blocking the effects of histamine, a chemical released during allergic reactions that can contribute to nasal congestion and other symptoms. Antihistamines can help reduce sneezing, itching, and runny nose. However, some antihistamines can cause drowsiness, so it is important to choose a non, sedating option if daytime alertness is a concern.

Expectorants: Expectorants are OTC medications that can help thin and loosen mucus in the respiratory passages, including the sinuses.

Nasal Sprays

Nasal Sprays: A Breath of Relief for Sinusitis

Sinusitis, a condition characterized by inflammation or infection of the sinuses, can cause a range of distressing symptoms. Nasal sprays are a common and convenient treatment option for sinusitis, providing targeted relief by delivering medication directly to the nasal passages. These sprays can help alleviate symptoms, reduce inflammation, and promote better airflow. Below we will delve into the intriguing world of nasal sprays, shedding light on their benefits, types, and considerations for effective use in the context of sinusitis.

Nasal sprays are topical medications delivered through a fine mist sprayed into the nostrils. They work by directly targeting the affected area, providing localized relief and reducing systemic side effects. Nasal sprays are available in various formulations and can contain different active ingredients, each serving a specific purpose in managing sinusitis symptoms.

Saline Nasal Sprays: Saline nasal sprays contain a sterile solution of salt and water. They are commonly used for nasal irrigation and moisturization. Saline sprays help rinse away mucus, allergens, and irritants, promoting sinus drainage and reducing nasal congestion. They are gentle, safe for regular use, and can be used by individuals of all ages, including children and pregnant women.

Decongestant Nasal Sprays: Decongestant nasal sprays provide temporary relief from nasal congestion by constricting the blood vessels in the nasal passages. They help reduce swelling and promote better airflow. Decongestant sprays should be used sparingly and for short periods (usually 3, 5 days) to avoid a rebound effect or dependency. Prolonged use can lead to a condition called rhinitis medicamentosa, where the nasal passages become dependent on the medication for relief.

Steroid Nasal Sprays: Steroid nasal sprays, also known as nasal corticosteroids, are effective in reducing inflammation in the nasal passages. They work by suppressing the immune response and reducing swelling. Steroid sprays are particularly beneficial for managing symptoms such as nasal congestion, runny nose, sneezing, and nasal itching. They are safe for long, term use and can provide significant relief for individuals with chronic sinusitis or allergic rhinitis.

Antihistamine Nasal Sprays: Antihistamine nasal sprays contain medications that block the effects of histamine, a chemical released during allergic reactions. They help reduce symptoms such as sneezing, itching, and runny nose caused by allergies or allergic rhinitis. Antihistamine sprays are especially useful when symptoms are localized to the nasal passages. It is important to note that some antihistamine sprays may cause drowsiness, so non, sedating options are available for individuals who need to remain alert during the day.

Combination Nasal Sprays: Combination nasal sprays often contain a combination of active ingredients, such as a steroid and an antihistamine. These sprays provide the benefits of both medications, targeting both inflammation and allergy symptoms. Combination sprays can be particularly beneficial for individuals with sinusitis triggered by allergies or those with persistent symptoms that do not respond to single, agent therapies.

When using nasal sprays for sinusitis, it is important to follow proper technique and guidelines for safe and effective use:

Prime the Spray: Before using a nasal spray for the first time or after a period of non, use, it is important to prime the spray as per the manufacturer's instructions. Priming involves activating the pump mechanism to ensure proper spray dispersion.

Decongestants

Decongestants: Unblocking the Path to Sinus Relief

Sinusitis, a condition characterized by inflammation or infection of the sinuses, can cause significant nasal congestion and discomfort. Decongestants are a popular and effective treatment option for relieving nasal congestion associated with sinusitis. These medications work by constricting the blood vessels in the nasal passages, reducing swelling and opening up the airways. Below we will delve into the intriguing world of decongestants, shedding light on their mechanism of action, types, considerations, and their role in managing sinusitis.

Decongestants work by targeting the blood vessels in the nasal passages. They come in different forms, including oral tablets, nasal sprays, and nasal drops. These medications contain active ingredients that stimulate receptors in the blood vessels, leading to constriction and reducing the blood flow to the nasal tissues. As a result, the swollen tissues shrink, providing relief from nasal congestion.

Oral Decongestants: Oral decongestants are available in tablet or liquid form and are commonly used to relieve nasal congestion caused by sinusitis. They work by constricting blood vessels throughout the body, including those in the nasal passages. This constriction reduces swelling and opens up the airways, allowing for easier breathing. Oral decongestants are typically short, acting and provide temporary relief. They are useful for managing acute symptoms but should be used with caution in individuals with certain medical conditions, such as high blood pressure or heart problems. It is important to read the instructions and consult a healthcare professional if there are any concerns.

Nasal Decongestant Sprays: Nasal decongestant sprays are a targeted approach for relieving nasal congestion associated with sinusitis. They contain decongestant medications that are sprayed directly into the nasal passages, delivering the medication to the affected area. Nasal sprays provide rapid relief by constricting the blood vessels in the nasal tissues, reducing swelling, and opening up the airways. These sprays can be effective in providing immediate relief from congestion, allowing for easier breathing. However, they should be used with caution and for short periods only, as prolonged use can lead to a rebound effect and worsen congestion. It is important to follow the instructions and not exceed the recommended usage duration.

Combination Decongestant Products: Some over, the, counter medications combine decongestants with other active ingredients to provide multi, symptom relief. These combination products often include antihistamines, pain relievers, or cough suppressants along with decongestants. They can provide relief not only from nasal congestion but also from associated symptoms such as headache, fever, or cough. Combination products are convenient for individuals experiencing multiple sinusitis symptoms. However, it is important to carefully read the labels, as some combination products may contain ingredients that are not suitable for certain individuals or may interact with other medications.

When using decongestants for sinusitis, it is important to consider the following:

Duration of Use: Decongestants, particularly nasal sprays, should be used for the shortest duration necessary to alleviate symptoms. Long, term or excessive use can lead to a condition called rhinitis medicamentosa, where the nasal passages become dependent on the medication for relief, and rebound congestion occurs when the medication is discontinued. To avoid this, it is recommended to use decongestant sprays for no longer than 3, 5 consecutive days.

Proper Administration: When using nasal sprays or drops, it is important to follow the instructions for proper administration. Shake the bottle well, tilt the head slightly forward, and insert the nozzle into one nostril while gently closing the other nostril with a finger.

Pain Relievers

Pain Relievers: Soothing the Aches and Pains of Sinusitis

Sinusitis, a condition characterized by inflammation or infection of the sinuses, can bring about uncomfortable symptoms, including facial pain, pressure, and headaches. Pain relievers are a common treatment option to alleviate these symptoms and provide much, needed relief. By targeting the underlying inflammation and reducing pain, these medications can help individuals manage the discomfort associated with sinusitis. Below we will explore the intriguing world of pain relievers in the context of sinusitis, shedding light on their mechanism of action, types, considerations, and their role in soothing the aches and pains of sinusitis.

Acetaminophen: Acetaminophen, commonly known as paracetamol, is a widely used over, the, counter pain reliever. It is effective in reducing pain and fever associated with sinusitis. Acetaminophen works by inhibiting the production of pain, causing substances in the body. It is generally well, tolerated and has fewer gastrointestinal side effects compared to nonsteroidal anti, inflammatory drugs (NSAIDs). However, it is important to follow the recommended dosage and not exceed the maximum daily limit to avoid potential liver toxicity.

Nonsteroidal Anti, inflammatory Drugs (NSAIDs): NSAIDs, such as ibuprofen and naproxen, are commonly used to relieve pain, reduce inflammation, and lower fever. They work by inhibiting the production of prostaglandins, chemicals that promote pain and inflammation. NSAIDs can provide effective relief for sinusitis, related symptoms, including facial pain, headaches, and fever. It is important to carefully read the instructions and follow the recommended dosage to minimize the risk of gastrointestinal side effects or other potential complications. Individuals with certain medical conditions, such as gastric ulcers or kidney problems, should consult a healthcare professional before using NSAIDs.

Combination Pain Relievers: Some over, the, counter medications combine pain relievers with other active ingredients to provide multi, symptom relief. These combination products often include decongestants, antihistamines, or cough suppressants along with pain relievers. They can provide relief not only from pain but also from associated symptoms such as nasal congestion, runny nose, or cough. Combination products are convenient for individuals experiencing multiple sinusitis symptoms. However, it is important to carefully read the labels and follow the instructions to ensure appropriate usage and avoid potential interactions or adverse effects.

Topical Analgesics: Topical analgesics, such as creams, gels, or patches, are applied directly to the skin over the affected area to provide localized pain relief. They can be helpful in relieving facial pain or headaches associated with sinusitis. Topical analgesics work by numbing the skin and underlying tissues, reducing pain signals. They can be particularly beneficial for individuals who prefer to avoid oral medications or have sensitivities to systemic pain relievers. It is important to follow the instructions for proper application and avoid using these products on broken or irritated skin.

Considerations and Precautions: While pain relievers can provide relief, it is important to use them judiciously and consider certain precautions:

a. Follow the Recommended Dosage: It is crucial to follow the recommended dosage instructions and not exceed the maximum daily limit. Taking more than the recommended dose can lead to adverse effects, including liver damage or gastrointestinal complications.

b. Read the Labels: Carefully reading the labels and understanding the active ingredients and potential side effects is essential. Some pain relievers may contain additional ingredients that may not be suitable for everyone or may interact with other medications.

Chapter Seven

Prescription Treatments

Prescription Treatments for Sinusitis: Unlocking the Power of Targeted Relief

Sinusitis, a condition characterized by inflammation or infection of the sinuses, can cause significant discomfort and disruption in daily life. While over, the, counter treatments can provide relief for many individuals, some cases of sinusitis may require prescription medications to effectively manage symptoms and promote healing. These prescription treatments offer a more targeted approach, addressing the underlying causes of sinusitis and providing specialized relief. Below we will explore the intriguing world of prescription treatments for sinusitis, shedding light on their mechanism of action, types, considerations, and their role in unlocking the power of targeted relief.

Antibiotics: Antibiotics are prescription medications used to treat bacterial sinusitis. When sinusitis is caused by a bacterial infection, antibiotics help eliminate the bacteria and clear the infection. These medications are usually prescribed when symptoms persist for more than 10 days, worsen after an initial improvement, or are severe from the onset. It is important to note that antibiotics are not effective against viral sinusitis, which is the more common form of the condition. Antibiotics should be taken as prescribed, and the full course of treatment should be completed to ensure the eradication of the infection and prevent the development of antibiotic resistance.

Nasal Corticosteroids: Nasal corticosteroids are prescription medications used to reduce inflammation in the nasal passages and sinuses. They are particularly beneficial for individuals with chronic or severe sinusitis. These medications work by suppressing the immune response and reducing swelling, thus alleviating symptoms such as nasal congestion, runny nose, and facial pain or pressure. Nasal corticosteroids are available in various formulations, including nasal sprays or drops. They are typically used on a daily basis for a prolonged period to achieve optimal results. It is important to follow the prescribed dosage and usage instructions, as well as any specific recommendations from the healthcare provider.

Oral Corticosteroids: In cases of severe or persistent sinusitis, oral corticosteroids may be prescribed for a short duration to provide relief and reduce inflammation. These medications are taken by mouth and work throughout the body to reduce inflammation, including in the sinuses. Oral corticosteroids are usually used when other treatments have not provided adequate relief or in situations where rapid symptom improvement is necessary. It is important to note that oral corticosteroids may have potential side effects, especially when used for extended periods, so they are typically prescribed for short durations under close medical supervision.

Antihistamines: Antihistamines are prescription medications used to relieve allergy, related symptoms associated with sinusitis. They work by blocking the effects of histamine, a chemical released during allergic reactions that can contribute to nasal congestion, sneezing, and itching. Prescription, strength antihistamines may be recommended for individuals with severe or persistent allergic rhinitis or sinusitis that is triggered by allergens. It is important to consult a healthcare professional to determine the most appropriate antihistamine for the specific condition and to understand potential side effects or drug interactions.

Leukotriene Modifiers: Leukotriene modifiers are prescription medications that block the action of leukotrienes, chemicals involved in the inflammatory response. They can be useful in managing symptoms of sinusitis, particularly when associated with conditions such as allergic rhinitis or asthma. Leukotriene modifiers can help reduce nasal congestion, inflammation, and other symptoms. They are typically prescribed when other treatments have not provided sufficient relief or in individuals with specific underlying conditions.

Immunotherapy: Immunotherapy, also known as allergy shots, may be recommended for individuals with sinusitis caused by allergies or recurring sinusitis triggered by allergens.

Antibiotics

Antibiotics: The Mighty Warriors Against Bacterial Sinusitis

Sinusitis, a condition characterized by inflammation or infection of the sinuses, can bring about significant discomfort and disruption in daily life. When sinusitis is caused by a bacterial infection, antibiotics emerge as powerful warriors in the fight against the invading bacteria. These prescription medications target the specific bacteria responsible for the infection, helping to clear the infection and alleviate symptoms. Below we will delve into the intriguing world of antibiotics in the context of sinusitis, shedding light on their mechanism of action, types, considerations, and their role in combating bacterial sinusitis.

Understanding Bacterial Sinusitis: Sinusitis can have various causes, including viruses, bacteria, and allergies. Bacterial sinusitis occurs when bacteria invade the sinuses, leading to an infection. It is important to distinguish between viral and bacterial sinusitis, as antibiotics are effective only against bacterial infections. Bacterial sinusitis is typically characterized by persistent symptoms lasting more than 10 days, severe symptoms from the onset, or symptoms that worsen after an initial improvement. In these cases, antibiotics are prescribed to target and eliminate the bacterial infection.

How Antibiotics Work: Antibiotics are medications that either kill bacteria (bactericidal) or inhibit their growth (bacteriostatic). They work by interfering with specific components or processes within the bacteria, ultimately leading to the disruption of their survival and reproduction. Different classes of antibiotics target different bacterial structures or mechanisms. For example, penicillins interfere with the synthesis of the bacterial cell wall, while macrolides inhibit bacterial protein synthesis.

Types of Antibiotics for Sinusitis: Several classes of antibiotics are commonly prescribed for bacterial sinusitis. The choice of antibiotic depends on various factors, including the suspected bacteria involved, local resistance patterns, individual patient factors, and allergy considerations. Commonly prescribed antibiotics for sinusitis include:

a. Penicillins: Penicillins, such as amoxicillin and amoxicillin, clavulanate, are commonly used as first, line treatment for sinusitis. They are effective against many types of bacteria and are well, tolerated by most individuals. However, overuse and misuse of penicillins have contributed to the emergence of antibiotic resistance.

b. Cephalosporins: Cephalosporins, such as cefuroxime and cefdinir, are another class of antibiotics commonly used in the treatment of sinusitis. They are effective against a broad spectrum of bacteria and are often prescribed as an alternative to penicillins for individuals with penicillin allergies.

c. Macrolides: Macrolides, such as azithromycin and clarithromycin, are a class of antibiotics that are often prescribed for individuals with allergies to penicillins or cephalosporins. They are effective against many types of bacteria, including some that may be resistant to other antibiotics. Macrolides are particularly useful for individuals with certain types of chronic or recurrent sinusitis.

d. Fluoroquinolones: Fluoroquinolones, such as levofloxacin and moxifloxacin, are broad, spectrum antibiotics that are reserved for more severe cases of sinusitis or when other antibiotics have not been effective. They are effective against a wide range of bacteria but are generally reserved for situations where other options have failed due to concerns about potential side effects and development of antibiotic resistance.

Considerations and Precautions: While antibiotics are powerful tools in combating bacterial sinusitis, it is important to use them judiciously and consider certain precautions:

a. Proper Diagnosis: Accurate diagnosis of bacterial sinusitis is crucial before initiating antibiotics. Inappropriate use of antibiotics,

Steroid Nasal Sprays

Steroid Nasal Sprays: A Breath of Relief for Sinusitis

Sinusitis, a condition characterized by inflammation or infection of the sinuses, can cause significant discomfort and impact one's quality of life. Nasal congestion, runny nose, facial pain, and pressure are common symptoms that can persist for extended periods. Steroid nasal sprays offer a breath of relief for individuals suffering from sinusitis. These prescription medications provide targeted anti, inflammatory action to reduce swelling, alleviate symptoms, and promote healing. Below we will explore the intriguing world of steroid nasal sprays in the context of sinusitis, shedding light on their mechanism of action, benefits, considerations, and their role in providing relief for sinusitis.

Understanding Sinusitis and Inflammation: Sinusitis occurs when the sinuses, hollow air, filled cavities within the facial bones, become inflamed or infected. Inflammation is the body's natural response to infection or irritation, and it causes the blood vessels in the sinuses to dilate, leading to swelling and increased mucus production. This inflammation can result in symptoms such as nasal congestion, facial pain, pressure, and difficulty breathing.

Mechanism of Action of Steroid Nasal Sprays: Steroid nasal sprays, also known as intranasal corticosteroids, work by reducing inflammation in the nasal passages and sinuses. These medications contain corticosteroids, which are synthetic versions of hormones naturally produced by the body. When sprayed directly into the nose, the corticosteroids bind to receptors in the nasal tissues and exert anti, inflammatory effects. This action helps to decrease swelling, reduce mucus production, and alleviate symptoms associated with sinusitis.

Benefits of Steroid Nasal Sprays: Steroid nasal sprays offer several benefits in managing sinusitis:

a. Targeted Relief: Steroid nasal sprays deliver medication directly to the inflamed nasal passages and sinuses, providing localized and targeted relief. This allows for a more effective reduction in inflammation compared to systemic medications that may have broader effects on the body.

b. Anti, inflammatory Action: The primary benefit of steroid nasal sprays is their potent anti, inflammatory action. By reducing inflammation, these sprays help to alleviate symptoms such as nasal congestion, runny nose, facial pain, and pressure.

c. Long, term Management: Steroid nasal sprays are effective for both short, term symptom relief and long, term management of chronic sinusitis. They can be used on a daily basis for an extended period to help control inflammation, prevent symptom flare, ups, and improve overall sinus health.

d. Minimal Systemic Side Effects: Unlike oral corticosteroids, which can have systemic side effects when taken in high doses or for prolonged periods, steroid nasal sprays have minimal systemic absorption. This reduces the risk of systemic side effects such as adrenal suppression or bone loss.

Considerations and Proper Use:

a. Prescription Requirement: Steroid nasal sprays are available by prescription only. It is important to consult a healthcare professional for an accurate diagnosis and appropriate prescription. They can evaluate the severity of sinusitis, identify the most suitable medication, and provide instructions for proper use.

b. Regular Use: Steroid nasal sprays are most effective when used consistently on a daily basis, even when symptoms improve. The full therapeutic effect may take several days to weeks to become apparent, so patience and regular use are key.

c. Proper Technique: To maximize the effectiveness of the spray, it is important to use the correct technique. Tilt the head slightly forward, insert the nozzle into one nostril, and spray while inhaling gently through the nose. Repeat the process for the other nostril. It is crucial to follow the instructions provided by the healthcare provider.

Immunotherapy

Immunotherapy: Empowering the Immune System in the Battle Against Sinusitis

Sinusitis, a condition characterized by inflammation or infection of the sinuses, can be a persistent and bothersome problem for many individuals. While medication and other treatments provide relief for some, others may find that their sinusitis is triggered by allergens or recurring infections. In such cases, immunotherapy offers a unique approach to tackle the underlying causes of sinusitis by empowering the immune system. Below we will explore the intriguing world of immunotherapy in relation to sinusitis, shedding light on its mechanism of action, benefits, considerations, and its role in empowering the immune system to fight against sinusitis.

Understanding Sinusitis and Allergic Triggers: Sinusitis can have various triggers, including allergens such as pollen, dust mites, pet dander, and mold. In individuals with allergic sinusitis, exposure to these allergens can lead to an exaggerated immune response, resulting in persistent inflammation of the sinuses. This allergic inflammation contributes to the symptoms associated with sinusitis, including nasal congestion, runny nose, sneezing, and facial pressure.

Mechanism of Action of Immunotherapy: Immunotherapy, also known as allergy shots or allergy immunotherapy, is a treatment approach that aims to desensitize the immune system to specific allergens. The treatment involves regular injections of a small amount of the allergen(s) to which the individual is allergic. The allergens are gradually increased in concentration over time, allowing the immune system to develop tolerance and reduce its overreaction to the allergens.

Benefits of Immunotherapy for Sinusitis:

a. Allergen, Specific Approach: Immunotherapy targets the specific allergens that trigger allergic sinusitis. By desensitizing the immune system to these allergens, the treatment addresses the root cause of the allergic inflammation, reducing the frequency and severity of sinusitis episodes.

b. Long, Term Symptom Relief: Immunotherapy aims to provide long, term relief by modifying the immune response to allergens. With continued treatment, individuals may experience a reduction in symptoms, decreased reliance on medications, and an improved overall quality of life.

c. Prevention of Progression: Allergic sinusitis can potentially progress to chronic sinusitis if left untreated. Immunotherapy can help prevent this progression by reducing the intensity of the allergic response and limiting the chronic inflammation that contributes to sinusitis.

d. Treatment Customization: Immunotherapy is tailored to each individual's specific allergies. Allergy testing is performed to identify the allergens to which the person is sensitized, and a personalized treatment plan is developed based on the results. This customization ensures that the treatment targets the specific allergens that trigger sinusitis symptoms in each individual.

Types of Immunotherapy:

a. Subcutaneous Immunotherapy (SCIT): Subcutaneous immunotherapy, or allergy shots, involves injecting small amounts of allergens under the skin. The injections are typically given once or twice a week initially, and then the frequency is gradually reduced as tolerance develops. SCIT requires regular visits to a healthcare provider for the administration of the injections.

b. Sublingual Immunotherapy (SLIT): Sublingual immunotherapy involves placing allergen extracts under the tongue. The allergens are absorbed through the oral mucosa, triggering an immune response. SLIT is often administered as tablets or drops, which can be taken at home. It offers the convenience of self, administration and eliminates the need for frequent healthcare visits.

Considerations and Precautions:

a. Suitability for Allergy, Induced Sinusitis: Immunotherapy is most suitable for individuals with allergic sinusitis, where specific allergens trigger symptoms.

Chapter Eight

Home Remedies and Lifestyle Changes

Home Remedies and Lifestyle Changes: Empowering Self, Care in Sinusitis Management

Sinusitis, a condition characterized by inflammation or infection of the sinuses, can cause significant discomfort and disrupt daily life. While medical treatments play a crucial role in managing sinusitis, there are also several home remedies and lifestyle changes that can provide relief and support the healing process. These natural approaches empower individuals to take an active role in managing their sinusitis symptoms. Below we will explore the intriguing world of home remedies and lifestyle changes in relation to sinusitis, shedding light on their benefits, considerations, and their role in empowering self, care in sinusitis management.

Nasal Irrigation: Nasal irrigation, also known as nasal wash or nasal saline rinse, involves flushing the nasal passages with a saline solution. This technique helps to moisturize the nasal passages, clear mucus, and remove irritants or allergens. Nasal irrigation can be performed using a neti pot, squeeze bottle, or nasal irrigation kit. It is important to use distilled or sterile water and follow proper hygiene practices to avoid contamination.

Steam Inhalation: Steam inhalation is a simple yet effective home remedy for sinusitis. Inhaling warm, moist air can help to soothe the nasal passages, relieve congestion, and facilitate drainage. To practice steam inhalation, fill a bowl with hot water, place a towel over the head to create a tent, and breathe in the steam for a few minutes. Adding essential oils, such as eucalyptus or peppermint, to the water can enhance the benefits. However, caution should be exercised to avoid burns or scalding.

Warm Compresses: Applying warm compresses to the face can help alleviate sinus pain and pressure. The warmth promotes blood circulation, reduces inflammation, and provides soothing relief. Simply soak a clean cloth in warm water, wring out the excess, and place it over the sinus areas, such as the forehead, cheeks, or nose. Repeat the process as needed for comfort and relief.

Hydration: Staying well, hydrated is essential for sinusitis management. Drinking an adequate amount of water and fluids helps to thin mucus, promote sinus drainage, and prevent congestion. Warm fluids, such as herbal teas or broths, can be particularly soothing. However, it is important to avoid excessive caffeine or alcohol consumption, as they can contribute to dehydration.

Humidification: Dry indoor air can worsen sinusitis symptoms, so using a humidifier can help to maintain proper humidity levels and prevent dryness. A humidifier adds moisture to the air, reducing nasal dryness, congestion, and irritation. It is important to clean the humidifier regularly to prevent the growth of mold or bacteria.

Rest and Sleep: Getting adequate rest and sleep is crucial for the body's healing processes. Rest allows the immune system to function optimally and supports the recovery from sinusitis. It is important to prioritize sleep hygiene by creating a comfortable sleeping environment, maintaining a consistent sleep schedule, and practicing relaxation techniques if needed.

Healthy Diet: A balanced and nutritious diet plays a vital role in overall health, including sinusitis management. Consuming a diet rich in fruits, vegetables, whole grains, lean proteins, and healthy fats provides essential nutrients and supports the immune system. Some foods, such as spicy foods or those high in histamines, may exacerbate sinusitis symptoms in some individuals, so it can be beneficial to identify and avoid trigger foods.

Allergen Management: For individuals with allergic sinusitis, minimizing exposure to allergens is crucial. This may involve implementing measures such as using allergen, proof covers on pillows and mattresses and regular cleaning to reduce dust and pet dander.

Hydration

Hydration: Quenching the Thirst of Sinusitis Relief

Sinusitis, a condition characterized by inflammation or infection of the sinuses, can bring about uncomfortable symptoms and disrupt daily life. While medical treatments are crucial for managing sinusitis, there is one simple and often overlooked remedy that can provide significant relief: hydration. Adequate hydration plays a vital role in promoting sinus health and alleviating sinusitis symptoms. Below we will delve into the intriguing world of hydration in relation to sinusitis, shedding light on its benefits, considerations, and its role in quenching the thirst for sinusitis relief.

Understanding Sinusitis and the Role of Hydration: Sinusitis occurs when the sinuses, air, filled cavities within the facial bones, become inflamed or infected. Proper hydration is essential for sinus health because it helps to thin mucus, promote efficient sinus drainage, and prevent congestion. When the body is well, hydrated, the nasal passages remain moist, allowing mucus to flow freely and prevent the accumulation of mucus and bacteria.

Benefits of Hydration for Sinusitis Relief:

a. Thinning of Mucus: Adequate hydration helps to thin the mucus in the nasal passages and sinuses, making it easier for mucus to drain. Thin mucus flows more freely, reducing the risk of blockages and congestion.

b. Promotion of Sinus Drainage: Hydration promotes the proper function of the cilia, tiny hair, like structures in the nasal passages that help move mucus and foreign particles out of the sinuses. Well, hydrated nasal passages allow the cilia to function optimally, facilitating the clearance of mucus and debris from the sinuses.

c. Prevention of Congestion: When the body is dehydrated, the nasal passages can become dry, leading to thickened mucus and congestion. Proper hydration helps to maintain the moisture levels in the nasal passages, preventing the development of dryness and congestion.

d. Support for the Immune System: Hydration plays a crucial role in supporting the immune system, which is responsible for fighting off infections and reducing inflammation. When the body is well, hydrated, the immune system functions optimally, enhancing its ability to combat infections and reduce inflammation in the sinuses.

Optimal Hydration Practices:

a. Drink Plenty of Water: Water is the best hydrating beverage and should be the primary source of hydration. It is recommended to drink at least 8 cups (64 ounces) of water per day, or more if needed. Sipping water throughout the day is more effective than consuming large quantities at once.

b. Herbal Teas and Warm Liquids: In addition to water, herbal teas and warm liquids can provide additional hydration and soothing benefits. Herbal teas, such as chamomile or peppermint, can help alleviate congestion and provide relief for sinusitis symptoms.

c. Avoid Dehydrating Beverages: Certain beverages, such as caffeinated drinks and alcohol, can contribute to dehydration. It is important to moderate the consumption of these beverages and balance them with an adequate intake of water.

d. Incorporate Hydrating Foods: Some foods have high water content and can contribute to hydration. Fruits and vegetables such as watermelon, cucumber, oranges, and celery are excellent choices for hydration.

Considerations for Optimal Hydration:

a. Individual Hydration Needs: The amount of water needed for optimal hydration varies from person to person and depends on various factors such as age, activity level, climate, and overall health. It is important to listen to the body's thirst cues and increase water intake during periods of increased activity or in hot weather.

Warm Compresses

Warm Compresses: Soothing Relief for Sinusitis Symptoms

Sinusitis, the inflammation or infection of the sinuses, can cause discomfort and disrupt daily life. The symptoms, including nasal congestion, facial pain, and pressure, can be bothersome and affect one's quality of life. While medical treatments play a crucial role in managing sinusitis, there is a simple and effective remedy that can provide soothing relief: warm compresses. Applying warmth to the affected areas can help alleviate sinusitis symptoms and promote healing. Below we will explore the intriguing world of warm compresses in relation to sinusitis, shedding light on their benefits, considerations, and their role in providing soothing relief.

Understanding Sinusitis and the Role of Warm Compresses: Sinusitis occurs when the sinuses, air, filled cavities within the facial bones, become inflamed or infected. Warm compresses, applied to the affected areas, can provide several benefits in managing sinusitis symptoms. The warmth helps to increase blood circulation, reduce inflammation, and provide a soothing effect, relieving nasal congestion, pain, and pressure.

Benefits of Warm Compresses for Sinusitis Relief:

a. Improved Blood Circulation: Applying warmth to the affected areas helps to dilate blood vessels, increasing blood flow to the sinuses. Improved blood circulation can aid in the delivery of oxygen and nutrients, promoting healing and reducing inflammation.

b. Reduction of Inflammation: Warm compresses help to reduce inflammation in the sinuses, alleviating symptoms such as nasal congestion, facial pain, and pressure. The warmth promotes the relaxation of muscles and tissues, easing discomfort and promoting a sense of relief.

c. Enhanced Sinus Drainage: Warm compresses can help to promote sinus drainage by thinning mucus and facilitating its movement out of the sinuses. This can relieve congestion and facilitate the clearing of the nasal passages.

d. Soothing Effect: The application of warmth can have a soothing effect on the affected areas, providing comfort and relaxation. It can help alleviate the discomfort associated with sinusitis and promote a sense of calmness.

How to Apply Warm Compresses for Sinusitis Relief:

a. Preparation: To apply a warm compress, start by soaking a clean cloth or towel in warm water. The water should be comfortably warm but not scalding. Wring out the excess water to avoid dripping.

b. Application: Place the warm compress over the affected areas, such as the forehead, cheeks, or nose, where the sinuses are located. Gently press the compress against the skin, ensuring it covers the entire area. Hold the compress in place for 10 to 15 minutes or until the compress begins to cool.

c. Repeat as Needed: Warm compresses can be applied multiple times a day, as needed, to provide relief. It is important to use a fresh warm compress for each application to maintain hygiene and effectiveness.

Considerations and Precautions:

a. Temperature: When preparing a warm compress, it is essential to ensure that the water is at a safe and comfortable temperature. Avoid using water that is too hot, as it can cause burns or skin damage. Test the temperature with your hand before applying the compress to the face.

b. Hygiene: To maintain proper hygiene, always use a clean cloth or towel for each warm compress application. This helps to prevent the spread of bacteria and reduce the risk of infection.

c. Combination with Other Treatments: Warm compresses can be used in conjunction with other sinusitis treatments, such as medication or nasal irrigation, to enhance their effectiveness. Consult a healthcare professional for guidance on integrating warm compresses into your overall sinusitis management plan.

Steam Inhalation

Steam Inhalation: A Soothing Vapor for Sinusitis Relief

Sinusitis, a condition characterized by inflammation or infection of the sinuses, can bring about uncomfortable symptoms and disrupt daily life. Nasal congestion, facial pain, and pressure are common complaints that individuals with sinusitis experience. While medical treatments are crucial for managing sinusitis, there is a simple and time, tested remedy that can provide soothing relief: steam inhalation. Inhaling warm, moist air can help alleviate sinusitis symptoms and promote healing. Below we will explore the intriguing world of steam inhalation in relation to sinusitis, shedding light on its benefits, considerations, and its role in providing soothing relief.

Understanding Sinusitis and the Role of Steam Inhalation: Sinusitis occurs when the sinuses, air, filled cavities within the facial bones, become inflamed or infected. Steam inhalation involves inhaling warm, moist air, which helps to soothe the nasal passages, reduce congestion, and promote sinus drainage. The warm vapor provides therapeutic benefits by moisturizing the nasal passages, loosening mucus, and relieving inflammation.

Benefits of Steam Inhalation for Sinusitis Relief:

a. Nasal Congestion Relief: Steam inhalation helps to alleviate nasal congestion by moisturizing and hydrating the nasal passages. The warm, moist air helps to loosen the mucus, making it easier to expel and reducing congestion.

b. Soothing Effect on Irritated Sinuses: The warmth of the steam can have a soothing effect on the inflamed sinuses, providing relief from facial pain, pressure, and discomfort. It helps to relax the muscles and tissues, easing tension and promoting a sense of relaxation.

c. Promotion of Sinus Drainage: Steam inhalation promotes sinus drainage by thinning the mucus and facilitating its movement out of the sinuses. This can help to relieve congestion, improve breathing, and reduce the risk of sinus infections.

d. Moisturization of the Nasal Passages: Dry nasal passages can exacerbate sinusitis symptoms. Steam inhalation provides moisture to the nasal passages, helping to prevent dryness and irritation. This can contribute to overall sinus health and reduce the frequency and severity of sinusitis episodes.

How to Perform Steam Inhalation for Sinusitis Relief:

a. Boil water: Start by boiling water in a pot or kettle until it reaches a rolling boil. It is important to use clean, filtered water to ensure the quality of the steam.

b. Transfer water to a bowl: Carefully pour the boiling water into a heat, resistant bowl. Place the bowl on a stable surface, such as a table or countertop.

c. Add essential oils (optional): For added benefits, you can add a few drops of essential oils to the hot water. Eucalyptus, peppermint, and tea tree oils are commonly used for their soothing and decongestant properties. However, it is important to use caution and follow the recommended dosage, as some essential oils can be irritating or cause allergies in certain individuals.

d. Create a tent: Lean over the bowl, creating a tent with a towel or large cloth, covering both your head and the bowl. This helps to trap the steam and direct it towards your face.

e. Inhale the steam: Close your eyes and inhale deeply through your nose, taking slow and steady breaths. Allow the warm, moist air to penetrate your nasal passages and sinuses. You can also breathe through your mouth if it feels more comfortable.

f. Duration of inhalation: Continue inhaling the steam for about 5, 10 minutes or as long as it remains comfortably warm.

Avoiding Irritants

Avoiding Irritants: Protecting Your Sinuses from Aggravation

Sinusitis, a condition characterized by inflammation or infection of the sinuses, can cause significant discomfort and disrupt daily life. Nasal congestion, facial pain, and pressure are common symptoms that individuals with sinusitis experience. While medical treatments are crucial for managing sinusitis, there are preventive measures individuals can take to minimize sinus irritation and reduce the risk of flare, ups. Avoiding irritants plays a key role in protecting the sinuses and maintaining sinus health. Below we will explore the intriguing world of avoiding irritants in relation to sinusitis, shedding light on their importance, common irritants to avoid, and their role in promoting sinus health.

Understanding Sinusitis and the Impact of Irritants: Sinusitis occurs when the sinuses, air, filled cavities within the facial bones, become inflamed or infected. Irritants, both environmental and lifestyle, related, can exacerbate sinusitis symptoms and contribute to ongoing inflammation. By avoiding these irritants, individuals can reduce the burden on their sinuses, minimize symptom severity, and support the healing process.

Common Irritants to Avoid for Sinusitis Relief:

a. Allergens: Allergens such as pollen, dust mites, pet dander, and mold can trigger allergic reactions and worsen sinusitis symptoms. To minimize exposure to allergens, individuals should:

Keep windows closed during high pollen seasons.

Use allergen, proof covers on pillows and mattresses to reduce exposure to dust mites.

Regularly clean carpets, rugs, and upholstery to remove pet dander and other allergens.

Maintain proper ventilation and humidity control to prevent the growth of mold.

b. Environmental Irritants: Various environmental factors can irritate the sinuses and contribute to inflammation. Individuals with sinusitis should be mindful of:

Air pollution: Avoid exposure to heavy traffic areas or industrial pollution as much as possible. Use air purifiers or filters to improve indoor air quality.

Strong odors and irritants: Steer clear of strong chemical odors, perfumes, cleaning products, and smoke, as these can irritate the nasal passages and sinuses.

c. Temperature and Humidity Extremes: Extreme temperature and humidity levels can impact sinus health. Individuals with sinusitis should:

Protect the nasal passages from cold, dry air by wearing scarves or using a humidifier to add moisture to indoor air.

Avoid sudden temperature changes and excessive exposure to cold weather.

d. Irritating Substances: Certain substances can irritate the nasal passages and sinuses, worsening sinusitis symptoms. Individuals should be cautious and avoid:

Irritant fumes: Steer clear of strong chemical fumes, cleaning products, paint, and other volatile substances that can irritate the sinuses.

Nasal irritants: Reduce the use of nasal sprays, decongestants, or other nasal medications that can lead to rebound congestion or nasal dryness when used excessively or for prolonged periods.

Importance of Avoiding Irritants for Sinusitis Relief:

a. Reduced Inflammation: By avoiding irritants, individuals can minimize inflammation in the sinuses, leading to reduced sinusitis symptoms such as congestion, pain, and pressure.

b. Prevention of Flare, ups: Irritants can trigger sinusitis flare, ups in susceptible individuals. By avoiding these triggers, individuals can reduce the frequency and severity of sinusitis episodes.

c. Enhanced Healing: By protecting the sinuses from irritants, individuals create a favorable environment for healing. This allows the body to recover from inflammation and infection, supporting the overall healing process.

Chapter Nine

Surgical Options

Surgical Options: Exploring Advanced Solutions for Sinusitis

Sinusitis, a condition characterized by inflammation or infection of the sinuses, can be a chronic and debilitating condition for some individuals. While medical treatments and lifestyle modifications can provide relief for many, there are cases where surgical intervention becomes necessary. Surgical options offer advanced solutions for managing sinusitis by addressing underlying structural issues, improving sinus drainage, and reducing the frequency and severity of symptoms. Below we will delve into the intriguing world of surgical options in relation to sinusitis, shedding light on their benefits, considerations, and their role in providing long, term relief.

Understanding Sinusitis and the Need for Surgical Intervention: Sinusitis occurs when the sinuses, air, filled cavities within the facial bones, become inflamed or infected. In some cases, sinusitis is not effectively managed by medical treatments alone. Persistent or recurrent sinusitis, structural abnormalities, or complications may indicate the need for surgical intervention to address the root cause of the condition.

Functional Endoscopic Sinus Surgery (FESS): Functional endoscopic sinus surgery is the most common surgical procedure performed for sinusitis. It is a minimally invasive technique that uses a thin, flexible tube with a camera (endoscope) to visualize and access the sinuses. The surgeon removes obstructing tissues, polyps, or bone spurs, opens blocked sinuses, and improves sinus drainage. FESS is effective in treating chronic sinusitis, nasal polyps, and structural abnormalities.

Balloon Sinuplasty: Balloon sinuplasty is a less invasive procedure that aims to open blocked sinuses using a small balloon catheter. The catheter is inserted into the sinus opening and then inflated to expand the sinus passage, allowing improved drainage. Balloon sinuplasty is a suitable option for individuals with chronic sinusitis who have not responded to medical treatments and prefer a minimally invasive approach.

Septoplasty: Septoplasty is a surgical procedure performed to correct a deviated septum, a condition where the nasal septum (the partition between the nostrils) is crooked or displaced. A deviated septum can obstruct sinus drainage, leading to chronic sinusitis. Septoplasty involves straightening or repositioning the septum, improving airflow and facilitating sinus drainage.

Turbinate Reduction: The turbinates are structures located on the sides of the nasal passages that help filter and humidify the air we breathe. In some cases, the turbinates can become enlarged or swollen, obstructing nasal airflow and contributing to sinusitis symptoms. Turbinate reduction is a surgical procedure that aims to decrease the size of the turbinates, improving nasal airflow and reducing congestion.

Ethmoidectomy: Ethmoidectomy is a surgical procedure specifically targeting the ethmoid sinuses, which are located between the eyes and nose. It involves the removal of infected or inflamed tissue within the ethmoid sinuses to improve drainage and reduce inflammation. Ethmoidectomy is often performed in conjunction with other sinus surgeries to address complex or severe cases of sinusitis.

Considerations and Precautions:

a. Candidacy for Surgery: Not all individuals with sinusitis require surgery. Surgical intervention is typically considered when other treatments have been ineffective or when structural abnormalities are present. A thorough evaluation by an ear, nose, and throat specialist is necessary to determine if surgery is appropriate.

b. Risks and Benefits: Like any surgical procedure, sinus surgery carries some risks, including bleeding, infection, scarring, and damage to surrounding structures. However, the potential benefits of improved sinus drainage, reduced symptoms, and enhanced quality of life often outweigh the risks.

Functional Endoscopic Sinus Surgery (FESS)

Functional Endoscopic Sinus Surgery (FESS): A Minimally Invasive Solution for Sinusitis Relief

Sinusitis, a condition characterized by inflammation or infection of the sinuses, can significantly impact one's quality of life. While medical treatments and lifestyle modifications provide relief for many individuals, there are cases where more advanced interventions are required. Functional Endoscopic Sinus Surgery (FESS) is a surgical procedure that offers a minimally invasive solution for managing chronic or recurrent sinusitis. Below we will explore the fascinating world of FESS, shedding light on its benefits, considerations, and its role in providing long, term relief for sinusitis.

Understanding Sinusitis and the Role of FESS: Sinusitis occurs when the sinuses, air, filled cavities within the facial bones, become inflamed or infected. In some cases, sinusitis is not effectively managed by medical treatments alone. FESS is a surgical procedure that aims to address the underlying structural issues contributing to sinusitis, allowing for improved sinus drainage and reduced inflammation.

The FESS Procedure: FESS is performed using an endoscope, a thin, flexible tube with a camera attached, which allows the surgeon to visualize and access the sinuses. The procedure is typically performed under general anesthesia or local anesthesia with sedation. The steps involved in FESS may include:

a. Diagnostic Evaluation: Before the surgery, a thorough evaluation is conducted to assess the severity and extent of sinus disease. Imaging studies, such as CT scans, are often used to aid in the diagnosis and surgical planning.

b. Sinus Access: The surgeon inserts the endoscope into the nasal cavity to visualize the sinuses. The procedure is guided by the images captured by the endoscope, which are displayed on a monitor.

c. Tissue Removal and Opening of Sinuses: Using specialized instruments, the surgeon removes obstructing tissues, such as polyps, nasal blockages, or thickened mucus, and opens up the blocked sinus passages. This allows for improved sinus drainage and ventilation.

d. Correction of Structural Abnormalities: If there are any structural abnormalities contributing to sinusitis, such as a deviated septum or nasal bone spurs, they can be addressed during the FESS procedure. The surgeon may straighten the septum or remove any obstructions to facilitate better airflow.

e. Balloon Sinuplasty (optional): In some cases, the FESS procedure may include balloon sinuplasty, a technique where a small balloon catheter is inserted into the sinus opening and inflated to widen the passage. This helps to further improve sinus drainage and ventilation.

Benefits of FESS for Sinusitis Relief:

a. Improved Sinus Drainage: FESS aims to restore normal sinus function by removing obstructions and opening blocked sinus passages. This allows for improved sinus drainage, reducing the risk of mucus buildup and subsequent infections.

b. Reduction of Symptoms: By addressing the underlying causes of sinusitis, FESS can significantly reduce symptoms such as nasal congestion, facial pain, pressure, and post, nasal drip. Many individuals experience a significant improvement in their overall quality of life after FESS.

c. Minimally Invasive Approach: FESS is a minimally invasive procedure, which means it is performed through the nostrils without the need for external incisions. This results in less scarring, minimal discomfort, and a shorter recovery time compared to traditional open surgeries.

d. Shorter Hospital Stay: FESS is typically performed on an outpatient basis, meaning that most individuals can go home on the same day as the surgery. This eliminates the need for an extended hospital stay, allowing for a quicker return to normal activities.

Balloon Sinuplasty

Balloon Sinuplasty: Expanding Horizons for Sinusitis Relief

Sinusitis, the inflammation or infection of the sinuses, can cause significant discomfort and affect one's quality of life. While medical treatments and lifestyle modifications provide relief for many individuals, there are cases where more advanced interventions are necessary. Balloon sinuplasty is a minimally invasive procedure that offers a revolutionary approach to managing chronic sinusitis. Below we will explore the fascinating world of balloon sinuplasty, shedding light on its benefits, considerations, and its role in providing long, term relief for sinusitis.

Understanding Sinusitis and the Need for Balloon Sinuplasty: Sinusitis occurs when the sinuses, air, filled cavities within the facial bones, become inflamed or infected. When sinusitis is chronic or does not respond well to medical treatments, balloon sinuplasty may be considered. This innovative procedure aims to open blocked sinus passages, improve drainage, and alleviate the symptoms of sinusitis.

The Balloon Sinuplasty Procedure: Balloon sinuplasty is a minimally invasive technique that uses a small balloon catheter to open blocked sinus passages. The procedure is typically performed in an outpatient setting and involves the following steps:

a. Anesthesia: Local or general anesthesia is administered to ensure patient comfort during the procedure. The choice of anesthesia depends on various factors, including patient preference and the surgeon's recommendation.

b. Balloon Insertion: A small, flexible balloon catheter is inserted into the blocked sinus passage through the nostril. The catheter is guided into the targeted area using endoscopic visualization, which provides real, time images of the sinuses.

c. Balloon Inflation: Once the balloon catheter is in position, it is gently inflated to expand the sinus opening. The inflation process is gradual and controlled to avoid excessive pressure on the sinus walls.

d. Sinus Passage Opening: The inflated balloon exerts pressure on the surrounding sinus tissues, causing them to widen and create a larger opening. This helps to improve sinus drainage and restore normal airflow.

e. Balloon Removal: After the desired sinus passage opening is achieved, the balloon is deflated and removed, leaving the newly opened sinus passage intact.

Benefits of Balloon Sinuplasty for Sinusitis Relief:

a. Minimally Invasive Approach: Balloon sinuplasty is considered a minimally invasive procedure because it does not require any cutting or removal of bone or tissue. This results in less trauma, reduced bleeding, and a faster recovery compared to traditional sinus surgery.

b. Improved Sinus Drainage: By expanding the sinus passages, balloon sinuplasty enhances sinus drainage, allowing mucus to flow freely and reducing the risk of congestion and infection. Improved sinus drainage can provide long, lasting relief from sinusitis symptoms.

c. Reduced Risk of Complications: Balloon sinuplasty carries a lower risk of complications compared to traditional sinus surgery. The procedure preserves the natural anatomy of the sinuses, minimizing the risk of scarring, structural changes, or post, operative discomfort.

d. Quicker Recovery Time: With balloon sinuplasty, the recovery time is typically shorter compared to traditional surgery. Most individuals can return to normal activities within a few days, experiencing minimal downtime and discomfort.

e. Customized Treatment: Balloon sinuplasty is a versatile procedure that can be tailored to each individual's specific needs. The technique can be applied to different sinuses and adjusted according to the severity of the condition, allowing for personalized treatment.

Image

,

Guided Surgery

Image, Guided Surgery: Navigating Precision for Sinusitis Relief

Sinusitis, the inflammation or infection of the sinuses, can cause significant discomfort and disrupt daily life. While medical treatments and minimally invasive procedures provide relief for many individuals, there are cases where more advanced interventions are required. Image, guided surgery is a groundbreaking technique that combines real, time imaging technology with surgical navigation systems to enhance precision and accuracy during sinus surgery. Below we will explore the fascinating world of image, guided surgery in relation to sinusitis, shedding light on its benefits, considerations, and its role in providing long, term relief.

Understanding Sinusitis and the Need for Image, Guided Surgery: Sinusitis occurs when the sinuses, air, filled cavities within the facial bones, become inflamed or infected. When sinusitis is complex, recurrent, or associated with structural abnormalities, image, guided surgery may be recommended. This advanced technique allows surgeons to navigate and visualize the intricate sinus anatomy, leading to more precise surgical outcomes.

The Basics of Image, Guided Surgery: Image, guided surgery involves the integration of real, time imaging technology and surgical navigation systems to provide accurate guidance during sinus procedures. The process typically involves the following steps:

a. Preoperative Imaging: Before surgery, imaging scans such as computed tomography (CT) or magnetic resonance imaging (MRI) are obtained to create detailed three, dimensional images of the sinuses. These images serve as a roadmap for the surgeon.

b. Registration: The preoperative images are registered or aligned with the patient's actual anatomy. This ensures that the virtual map corresponds accurately to the patient's unique sinus structures.

c. Surgical Navigation System: During surgery, a surgical navigation system is used to track the position of surgical instruments in real, time relative to the patient's anatomy. This system provides continuous feedback, enabling the surgeon to visualize their instruments within the sinus cavities.

d. Visualization and Guidance: The surgeon can view the real, time images on a monitor, overlaid with the patient's anatomy and the precise location of the surgical instruments. This helps guide the surgeon in performing precise and targeted maneuvers during the procedure.

Benefits of Image, Guided Surgery for Sinusitis Relief:

a. Enhanced Precision: Image, guided surgery allows for precise localization of sinus structures and abnormalities, reducing the risk of accidental damage to critical structures such as nerves, blood vessels, or the skull base. This precision helps to optimize surgical outcomes and minimize post, operative complications.

b. Accurate Sinus Mapping: Image, guided surgery provides an accurate and detailed map of the sinuses, enabling the surgeon to identify and address specific areas of inflammation, infection, or structural abnormalities. This targeted approach improves the effectiveness of the surgical intervention.

c. Complex Cases: Image, guided surgery is particularly valuable in complex cases where there is extensive inflammation, scarring, or previous surgical interventions. It allows the surgeon to navigate through challenging anatomy and increase the success rate of the procedure.

d. Reduced Invasiveness: By enhancing precision, image, guided surgery can potentially reduce the invasiveness of the procedure. With a more targeted approach, the surgeon can minimize tissue trauma and optimize the preservation of healthy sinus structures.

e. Improved Outcomes: The enhanced accuracy and precision provided by image, guided surgery contribute to improved surgical outcomes. This can lead to better symptom relief, reduced risk of recurrence, and an overall improvement in the patient's quality of life.

Considerations and Precautions:

a. Surgical Expertise: Image, guided surgery requires specialized training and expertise. It is essential to choose a surgeon who is experienced in utilizing the technology and has a thorough understanding of sinus anatomy and surgical techniques.

Chapter Ten

Post, Surgery Care and Recovery

Post, Surgery Care and Recovery: Nurturing Sinus Health after Surgery

Sinusitis, the inflammation or infection of the sinuses, can be a chronic and debilitating condition. When medical treatments and other interventions fail to provide relief, sinus surgery may be recommended. However, the journey towards sinusitis relief doesn't end with the surgical procedure. Post, surgery care and recovery play a crucial role in ensuring optimal healing, minimizing complications, and promoting long, term sinus health. Below we will explore the essential aspects of post, surgery care and recovery in relation to sinusitis, shedding light on their significance, considerations, and their role in nurturing sinus health.

Understanding Sinus Surgery and the Importance of Post, Surgery Care: Sinus surgery is performed to address structural abnormalities, improve sinus drainage, and alleviate symptoms of sinusitis. While surgery can provide significant relief, proper post, surgery care is vital for optimal healing and long, term success. It aims to reduce the risk of complications, support the healing process, and maintain sinus health.

Nasal Irrigation: Nasal irrigation, also known as nasal rinsing or nasal lavage, is a common practice recommended after sinus surgery. It involves flushing the nasal passages with a saline solution to remove mucus, debris, and promote healing. Nasal irrigation can help:

a. Keep the nasal passages moist: Proper hydration of the nasal passages can reduce discomfort, prevent crusting, and support healing.

b. Clear mucus and debris: Nasal irrigation helps remove mucus, blood clots, and debris that may accumulate after surgery. This promotes better airflow and reduces the risk of infection.

c. Reduce congestion and swelling: By reducing congestion and swelling, nasal irrigation can improve breathing and relieve discomfort.

Pain Management: Pain and discomfort are common after sinus surgery. Effective pain management strategies are essential for a smooth recovery. These may include:

a. Medications: Pain medications prescribed by the surgeon can help manage post, operative pain. It is crucial to follow the prescribed dosage and schedule.

b. Cold compresses: Applying cold compresses to the face can help alleviate pain and reduce swelling. Ensure that the compress is wrapped in a cloth to avoid direct contact with the skin.

c. Head elevation: Sleeping with the head elevated can minimize congestion, promote better drainage, and reduce pain and swelling.

Wound Care and Nasal Packing: Depending on the type of sinus surgery performed, nasal packing may be placed inside the nasal passages to control bleeding and provide support. It is essential to follow the surgeon's instructions regarding the care and removal of nasal packing. Proper wound care includes:

a. Cleaning the incision site: If there are external incisions, it is crucial to keep the area clean and dry as per the surgeon's instructions.

b. Avoiding excessive nose blowing: Vigorous nose blowing can disrupt healing and cause bleeding. Gentle blowing or using saline nasal sprays can help clear the nasal passages without excessive force.

c. Nasal saline sprays: Saline nasal sprays or mists can provide moisture to the nasal passages, promote healing, and prevent crusting.

Follow, up Appointments: Regular follow, up appointments with the surgeon are essential for monitoring healing progress, managing any complications, and addressing any concerns or questions. These appointments may include:

a. Evaluation of healing: The surgeon will assess the healing process and determine if any further interventions are necessary.

b. Removal of nasal packing: If nasal packing was used, the surgeon will remove it during a follow, up visit. This process is typically done painlessly and should be performed by a healthcare professional.

Expectations and Recovery Time

Expectations and Recovery Time: Navigating the Road to Recovery from Sinus Surgery

Sinusitis, a condition characterized by inflammation or infection of the sinuses, can significantly impact one's quality of life. When medical treatments fail to provide relief, sinus surgery may be recommended. However, it is important to have realistic expectations and understand the recovery process involved. Below we will explore the expectations and recovery time associated with sinus surgery, shedding light on the factors that influence recovery, milestones in the healing journey, and tips for a smooth recovery.

Understanding Sinus Surgery and Recovery: Sinus surgery is performed to address structural abnormalities, improve sinus drainage, and alleviate symptoms of sinusitis. Recovery from sinus surgery involves a healing process that varies from individual to individual. It is important to note that while sinus surgery can provide significant relief, the full benefits may not be immediately apparent, and complete recovery may take time.

Factors Affecting Recovery Time:

a. Type of Surgery: The specific type of sinus surgery performed can influence the recovery time. For example, minimally invasive procedures such as balloon sinuplasty or endoscopic surgery generally have shorter recovery periods compared to more extensive procedures like open sinus surgery.

b. Individual Healing Ability: Each person's body responds differently to surgery and heals at its own pace. Factors such as age, overall health, and immune system function can affect the speed of recovery.

c. Severity of Sinusitis: The severity of sinusitis prior to surgery can impact the recovery time. Chronic or long, standing sinusitis may require a longer recovery period compared to acute or less severe cases.

d. Adherence to Post, Operative Instructions: Following post, operative care instructions provided by the surgeon is crucial for a successful recovery. Compliance with medication, wound care, and lifestyle recommendations can positively influence the healing process.

Immediate Post, Surgery Expectations:

a. Discomfort and Pain: It is normal to experience some discomfort, pain, and swelling immediately after sinus surgery. The level of pain can vary depending on the extent of the surgery and individual pain tolerance. Pain medication prescribed by the surgeon can help manage these symptoms.

b. Nasal Congestion and Drainage: Nasal congestion and drainage are common after sinus surgery. This is a natural part of the healing process as the body adjusts to the changes made during surgery. Nasal saline sprays or rinses can help alleviate congestion and promote healing.

c. Fatigue: Fatigue is common during the initial recovery period. The body requires energy to heal, and rest is essential for a smooth recovery. Adequate sleep and avoiding strenuous activities can help combat fatigue.

d. Nasal Packing (if applicable): If nasal packing was used during surgery, it will be removed during a follow, up appointment. Nasal packing can cause temporary discomfort but provides support and helps control bleeding during the early stages of healing.

Milestones in the Recovery Journey:

a. First Week: The first week after surgery is crucial for initial healing. Nasal congestion, drainage, and mild discomfort are expected during this period. It is important to follow post, operative care instructions, including proper wound care, pain medication usage, and avoiding activities that can increase the risk of complications.

b. Two to Three Weeks: During this time, gradual improvements in symptoms can be observed. Nasal congestion and drainage may decrease, and breathing becomes easier. However, it is essential to avoid strenuous activities and follow the surgeon's guidance for a smooth recovery.

c. Four to Six Weeks: Most individuals experience significant improvement in their symptoms within four to six weeks after surgery. Swelling and inflammation continue to decrease, allowing for better sinus drainage and improved breathing.

Post

,

Surgery Care

Post, Surgery Care: Nurturing Sinus Health for Optimal Recovery

Sinusitis, the inflammation or infection of the sinuses, can significantly impact one's quality of life. When medical treatments fail to provide relief, sinus surgery may be recommended. However, the journey to sinusitis relief doesn't end with the surgical procedure. Post, surgery care plays a crucial role in ensuring optimal healing, minimizing complications, and nurturing long, term sinus health. Below we will explore the essential aspects of post, surgery care in relation to sinusitis, shedding light on their significance, considerations, and their role in nurturing sinus health.

Understanding Sinus Surgery and the Importance of Post, Surgery Care: Sinus surgery is performed to address structural abnormalities, improve sinus drainage, and alleviate symptoms of sinusitis. While surgery can provide significant relief, proper post, surgery care is vital for optimal healing and long, term success. It aims to reduce the risk of complications, support the healing process, and maintain sinus health.

Pain Management: Pain and discomfort are common after sinus surgery. Effective pain management strategies are essential for a smooth recovery. These may include:

a. Medications: Pain medications prescribed by the surgeon can help manage post, operative pain. It is crucial to follow the prescribed dosage and schedule.

b. Cold Compresses: Applying cold compresses to the face can help alleviate pain and reduce swelling. Ensure that the compress is wrapped in a cloth to avoid direct contact with the skin.

c. Head Elevation: Sleeping with the head elevated can minimize congestion, promote better drainage, and reduce pain and swelling.

Nasal Irrigation: Nasal irrigation, also known as nasal rinsing or nasal lavage, is a common practice recommended after sinus surgery. It involves flushing the nasal passages with a saline solution to remove mucus, debris, and promote healing. Nasal irrigation can help:

a. Keep the Nasal Passages Moist: Proper hydration of the nasal passages can reduce discomfort, prevent crusting, and support healing.

b. Clear Mucus and Debris: Nasal irrigation helps remove mucus, blood clots, and debris that may accumulate after surgery. This promotes better airflow and reduces the risk of infection.

c. Reduce Congestion and Swelling: By reducing congestion and swelling, nasal irrigation can improve breathing and relieve discomfort.

Wound Care and Nasal Packing: Depending on the type of sinus surgery performed, nasal packing may be placed inside the nasal passages to control bleeding and provide support. It is essential to follow the surgeon's instructions regarding the care and removal of nasal packing. Proper wound care includes:

a. Cleaning the Incision Site: If there are external incisions, it is crucial to keep the area clean and dry as per the surgeon's instructions.

b. Avoiding Excessive Nose Blowing: Vigorous nose blowing can disrupt healing and cause bleeding. Gentle blowing or using saline nasal sprays can help clear the nasal passages without excessive force.

c. Nasal Saline Sprays: Saline nasal sprays or mists can provide moisture to the nasal passages, promote healing, and prevent crusting.

Medication Management:

a. Antibiotics: In some cases, antibiotics may be prescribed after sinus surgery to prevent infection or treat any existing infection. It is important to take the full course of antibiotics as prescribed by the surgeon.

b. Steroid Nasal Sprays: Steroid nasal sprays are commonly prescribed to reduce inflammation and promote healing. It is important to follow the instructions for proper usage and continue using them as directed.

c. Pain Medications: Pain medications may be prescribed to manage post, operative pain. It is essential to follow the prescribed dosage.

Risks and Complications

Risks and Complications: Navigating the Path to Sinus Surgery Safety

Sinusitis, the inflammation or infection of the sinuses, can cause significant discomfort and affect one's quality of life. When medical treatments and other interventions fail to provide relief, sinus surgery may be recommended. While sinus surgery can offer significant benefits, it is important to be aware of the potential risks and complications associated with the procedure. Below we will explore the risks and complications related to sinus surgery, shedding light on their significance, considerations, and steps to minimize their occurrence.

Understanding Sinus Surgery and the Need for Risk Assessment: Sinus surgery is performed to address structural abnormalities, improve sinus drainage, and alleviate symptoms of sinusitis. Before undergoing surgery, a thorough evaluation is conducted to assess the individual's candidacy and identify potential risk factors. It is crucial to have open and honest communication with the surgeon, discussing any pre, existing conditions, allergies, or previous surgical experiences.

General Risks and Complications:

a. Bleeding: Bleeding is a common risk associated with sinus surgery. While surgeons take precautions to minimize bleeding during the procedure, it can occur during the surgery or in the post, operative period. If excessive bleeding occurs, it may require intervention such as nasal packing or cauterization to control it.

b. Infection: As with any surgical procedure, there is a risk of infection after sinus surgery. The surgeon may prescribe antibiotics to minimize this risk. It is important to closely follow the prescribed medication regimen and report any signs of infection, such as increased pain, swelling, or discharge.

c. Adverse Reaction to Anesthesia: Anesthesia is used during sinus surgery to ensure patient comfort and safety. However, there is always a small risk of adverse reactions to anesthesia. The anesthesiologist will evaluate the patient's medical history and take appropriate measures to minimize this risk.

d. Scarring: Sinus surgery involves making incisions in the nasal passages and potentially removing or reshaping tissues. While surgeons strive to minimize scarring, some degree of scarring may occur. It is important to follow post, operative care instructions to promote optimal healing and minimize scarring.

Specific Risks and Complications:

a. Damage to Surrounding Structures: During sinus surgery, there is a small risk of unintentional damage to surrounding structures such as the eye, brain, blood vessels, or nerves. Surgeons take precautions, such as using imaging technology or intraoperative monitoring, to minimize this risk. It is essential to choose a skilled and experienced surgeon to further reduce this possibility.

b. Recurrence of Sinusitis: Sinus surgery aims to improve sinus drainage and alleviate symptoms of sinusitis. However, there is a chance that sinusitis may recur or persist despite surgery. This may be due to underlying factors such as ongoing inflammation, structural abnormalities, or underlying medical conditions.

c. Nasal Obstruction: In some cases, sinus surgery may result in nasal obstruction. This can occur due to scar tissue formation or inadequate healing of the nasal passages. Additional interventions or revision surgery may be necessary to address nasal obstruction if it occurs.

d. Changes in Smell or Taste: Following sinus surgery, some individuals may experience temporary or permanent changes in their sense of smell or taste. These changes are generally rare and may resolve over time. It is important to discuss any concerns with the surgeon if such changes occur.

Minimizing Risks and Complications:

a. Choosing a Skilled Surgeon: The choice of surgeon plays a significant role in minimizing risks and complications. A skilled and experienced surgeon with a proven track record in sinus surgery can offer a higher level of safety and expertise.

Chapter Eleven

Prevention Strategies

Prevention Strategies: Safeguarding Sinus Health and Preventing Sinusitis

Sinusitis, the inflammation or infection of the sinuses, can cause significant discomfort and disrupt daily life. While medical treatments and surgical interventions offer relief, prevention strategies play a crucial role in safeguarding sinus health and reducing the risk of sinusitis. By adopting proactive measures, individuals can minimize their susceptibility to sinusitis and maintain optimal sinus health. Below we will explore effective prevention strategies in relation to sinusitis, shedding light on their significance, considerations, and practical steps to incorporate into daily life.

Understanding Sinusitis and the Importance of Prevention: Sinusitis occurs when the sinuses become inflamed or infected, often due to factors such as allergies, viral or bacterial infections, or structural abnormalities. Prevention strategies aim to reduce the risk of sinusitis by addressing these underlying causes and promoting overall sinus health.

Maintain Good Nasal Hygiene:

a. Nasal Irrigation: Regular nasal irrigation with saline solution can help remove irritants, allergens, and excess mucus from the nasal passages. This practice can promote proper sinus drainage and reduce the likelihood of infection.

b. Proper Hand Hygiene: Regular handwashing with soap and water, especially before touching the face or nose, can prevent the spread of bacteria and viruses that can cause sinusitis.

c. Avoid Irritants: Minimize exposure to irritants such as cigarette smoke, strong chemicals, and environmental pollutants. These substances can irritate the nasal passages and increase the risk of sinus inflammation.

Manage Allergies:

a. Identify Triggers: If you have allergies, work with a healthcare professional to identify specific allergens that trigger your symptoms. Common allergens include pollen, dust mites, pet dander, and mold.

b. Allergen Avoidance: Take steps to minimize exposure to identified allergens. Keep indoor spaces clean and well, ventilated, use allergy, proof bedding, and consider using air purifiers to reduce allergen levels.

c. Allergy Medications: If necessary, use allergy medications as prescribed by your healthcare provider to control allergy symptoms and reduce the risk of sinusitis.

Boost Immune System:

a. Healthy Diet: Maintain a balanced diet rich in fruits, vegetables, whole grains, and lean proteins. These foods provide essential nutrients and antioxidants that support a robust immune system.

b. Regular Exercise: Engage in regular physical activity to promote overall health and strengthen the immune system. Aim for at least 150 minutes of moderate, intensity exercise per week.

c. Adequate Sleep: Prioritize quality sleep to ensure proper immune system function. Aim for 7, 9 hours of uninterrupted sleep each night.

d. Stress Management: Chronic stress can weaken the immune system. Incorporate stress management techniques such as meditation, deep breathing exercises, or engaging in activities you enjoy.

Maintain Healthy Sinus Environment:

a. Humidify the Air: Dry air can irritate the nasal passages and increase the risk of sinusitis. Use a humidifier to maintain a comfortable level of humidity in your home, especially during dry seasons.

b. Avoid Nasal Irritants: Minimize exposure to substances that can irritate the nasal passages, such as strong perfumes, cleaning chemicals, and harsh hair sprays.

c. Quit Smoking: Smoking damages the respiratory system and impairs the function of the sinuses. If you smoke, consider quitting to reduce the risk of sinusitis and improve overall health.

Regular Dental Care:

a. Oral Hygiene: Maintain good oral hygiene by brushing your teeth at least twice a day and flossing daily. Poor oral health can contribute to the development of sinus infections.

Regular Hygiene

Regular Hygiene: A Key Element in Sinus Health and Prevention of Sinusitis

Sinusitis, the inflammation or infection of the sinuses, can cause significant discomfort and disrupt daily life. While medical treatments and preventive strategies play a crucial role in managing sinusitis, regular hygiene practices are equally important in maintaining sinus health and reducing the risk of sinusitis. By incorporating simple yet effective hygiene habits into our daily routines, we can promote optimal sinus health and minimize the chances of sinus, related issues. Below we will explore the significance of regular hygiene in relation to sinusitis, shedding light on practical steps and considerations for maintaining sinus health.

Understanding Sinusitis and the Role of Hygiene: Sinusitis occurs when the sinuses become inflamed or infected, often due to factors such as allergies, viral or bacterial infections, or structural abnormalities. Regular hygiene practices aim to reduce the risk of sinusitis by addressing these underlying causes and promoting overall sinus health.

Nasal Hygiene:

a. Nasal Washing: Regular nasal washing with saline solution can help remove irritants, allergens, and excess mucus from the nasal passages. This practice aids in maintaining clear and healthy sinuses, reducing the risk of infection and inflammation.

b. Proper Hand Hygiene: Good hand hygiene is essential in preventing the spread of bacteria and viruses that can cause sinusitis. Wash your hands thoroughly with soap and water for at least 20 seconds before touching your face, especially your nose.

c. Avoid Irritants: Minimize exposure to irritants such as cigarette smoke, strong chemicals, and environmental pollutants. These substances can irritate the nasal passages, leading to inflammation and an increased risk of sinusitis.

Oral Hygiene:

a. Regular Brushing: Brush your teeth at least twice a day, using a soft, bristled toothbrush and fluoride toothpaste. Proper oral hygiene helps prevent oral infections that can spread to the sinuses and contribute to sinusitis.

b. Flossing: Flossing daily helps remove food particles and bacteria from between the teeth and along the gumline. By preventing gum disease and tooth decay, you can reduce the risk of sinus infections.

c. Tongue Cleaning: Use a tongue scraper or gently brush your tongue to remove bacteria and debris that can contribute to bad breath and oral infections. Maintaining a clean tongue helps maintain overall oral health.

Environmental Hygiene:

a. Clean Living Spaces: Regularly clean and vacuum your living spaces to reduce the presence of dust, pet dander, mold spores, and other allergens. Use high, efficiency particulate air (HEPA) filters in vacuum cleaners and air purifiers to remove airborne allergens effectively.

b. Bedding and Pillow Care: Wash your bedding regularly in hot water to eliminate dust mites and allergens. Additionally, consider using allergen, proof pillow covers to reduce exposure to dust mites and prevent potential allergic reactions.

c. Humidity Control: Maintain a comfortable level of humidity in your home. High humidity can promote the growth of mold and dust mites, while low humidity can dry out the nasal passages. Use a humidifier or dehumidifier to maintain an optimal humidity level.

Personal Hygiene:

a. Avoid Sharing Personal Items: To reduce the risk of bacterial or viral infections, avoid sharing personal items such as towels, tissues, nasal sprays, or makeup applicators. These items can harbor bacteria or viruses that may contribute to sinusitis.

b. Regular Handwashing: Wash your hands thoroughly and frequently, especially before eating, after using the restroom, or when coming into contact with surfaces that may be contaminated. Proper handwashing helps prevent the spread of germs that can cause sinus infections.

Humidifiers

Humidifiers: The Power of Moisture in Sinus Health and Management of Sinusitis

Sinusitis, the inflammation or infection of the sinuses, can cause discomfort and disrupt daily life. While medical treatments and preventive strategies play a crucial role in managing sinusitis, the use of humidifiers can significantly contribute to sinus health and help alleviate sinus, related symptoms. By adding moisture to the air we breathe, humidifiers can create an optimal environment for the sinuses, promoting comfort and reducing the risk of sinusitis. Below we will explore the significance of humidifiers in relation to sinus health, shedding light on their benefits, considerations, and practical tips for using them effectively.

Understanding Sinusitis and the Role of Humidity: Sinusitis occurs when the sinuses become inflamed or infected, often due to factors such as allergies, viral or bacterial infections, or structural abnormalities. Humidity, or the moisture content in the air, plays a crucial role in sinus health by keeping the nasal passages moist, promoting proper sinus drainage, and preventing dryness and irritation.

How Humidifiers Work:

a. Adding Moisture: Humidifiers are devices designed to increase the moisture content in the air. They emit water vapor or steam into the surrounding environment, raising the humidity level and creating a more comfortable and sinus, friendly atmosphere.

b. Types of Humidifiers: There are several types of humidifiers available, including evaporative humidifiers, ultrasonic humidifiers, warm mist humidifiers, and cool mist humidifiers. Each type has its own advantages and considerations, and choosing the right one depends on personal preferences and specific needs.

Benefits of Humidifiers for Sinus Health:

a. Relief from Dryness: Dry air can cause dryness and irritation in the nasal passages, leading to discomfort and increased susceptibility to sinusitis. Humidifiers add moisture to the air, alleviating dryness and promoting a soothing environment for the sinuses.

b. Sinus Drainage Support: Proper sinus drainage is essential for flushing out mucus and preventing congestion. By maintaining optimal humidity levels, humidifiers help keep the nasal passages moist and facilitate efficient sinus drainage.

c. Soothing Congestion: Humidity can help relieve nasal congestion by moisturizing the nasal passages and reducing inflammation. This can provide relief from symptoms such as stuffiness, pressure, and difficulty breathing.

d. Thinner Mucus Secretions: Dry air can lead to thickened mucus secretions, making it harder for the sinuses to drain properly. Humidifiers promote thinner mucus consistency, aiding in easier expulsion and reducing the risk of sinus blockage and infection.

Considerations when Using Humidifiers:

a. Optimal Humidity Level: The ideal humidity level for sinus health is generally between 40% to 60%. Higher humidity levels may promote the growth of mold, dust mites, or bacteria, while excessively low humidity can still cause dryness and discomfort.

b. Regular Cleaning: To prevent the growth of mold, bacteria, or other pathogens, it is crucial to clean and maintain the humidifier regularly. Follow the manufacturer's instructions for cleaning and disinfection, and replace filters or cartridges as recommended.

c. Distilled or Filtered Water: Using distilled or filtered water in the humidifier can help minimize the buildup of minerals or impurities, preventing the release of airborne particles that may irritate the sinuses.

d. Proper Placement: Place the humidifier in an appropriate location to maximize its effectiveness. It should be positioned on a flat surface away from walls and furniture, ensuring proper air circulation and avoiding any potential hazards or damage.

Avoiding Allergens

Avoiding Allergens: Shielding Sinus Health from Allergic Triggers

Sinusitis, the inflammation or infection of the sinuses, can cause significant discomfort and disrupt daily life. While medical treatments and preventive measures play a vital role in managing sinusitis, avoiding allergens is a key strategy in preventing allergic reactions and reducing the risk of sinus, related issues. By minimizing exposure to allergens, individuals can protect their sinus health, alleviate symptoms, and maintain a higher quality of life. Below we will explore the significance of avoiding allergens in relation to sinusitis, shedding light on common allergens, considerations, and practical steps to minimize their impact.

Understanding Sinusitis and Allergens: Sinusitis can be triggered or aggravated by allergens, substances that cause an allergic reaction in susceptible individuals. Common allergens include pollen, dust mites, pet dander, mold spores, and certain foods. By avoiding or reducing exposure to these allergens, individuals can lower their risk of developing sinusitis or experiencing allergic reactions that worsen existing sinus conditions.

Identifying Common Allergens:

a. Pollen: Pollen from trees, grasses, and weeds is a prevalent allergen, especially during specific seasons. Monitor local pollen counts and limit outdoor activities during peak pollen times. Keep windows closed and use air purifiers or pollen filters in the home.

b. Dust Mites: These microscopic organisms thrive in bedding, carpets, upholstery, and stuffed toys. Encase mattresses and pillows in allergen, proof covers, wash bedding in hot water regularly, and vacuum frequently using a high, efficiency particulate air (HEPA) filter to minimize dust mite exposure.

c. Pet Dander: Animal fur, skin flakes, and saliva can trigger allergies. If you're allergic, consider keeping pets out of the bedroom and frequently vacuuming upholstered furniture and carpets. Regularly groom and bathe pets to reduce dander buildup.

d. Mold Spores: Mold thrives in damp environments, such as bathrooms, kitchens, and basements. Keep these areas well, ventilated, repair any leaks or water damage promptly, and use mold inhibitors or dehumidifiers to control moisture levels.

e. Food Allergens: Some individuals may experience sinus symptoms due to specific food allergies. Common culprits include dairy products, gluten, shellfish, nuts, and eggs. If you suspect a food allergy, consult with a healthcare professional for allergy testing and dietary guidance.

Practical Steps to Avoid Allergens:

a. Monitor Allergy Forecasts: Stay informed about local allergy forecasts, which provide information about the current pollen levels and common triggers. Adjust your activities and travel plans accordingly to minimize exposure during high, allergy periods.

b. Maintain Clean Indoor Air: Regularly clean and vacuum your living spaces to minimize dust and pet dander. Use vacuum cleaners equipped with HEPA filters to trap small particles effectively. Consider using air purifiers with HEPA filters to further improve indoor air quality.

c. Create an Allergen, Free Bedroom: Keep the bedroom a safe haven by implementing allergen, reducing strategies. Use hypoallergenic bedding, wash bedding in hot water weekly, and limit the presence of carpets and upholstered furniture that can harbor dust mites and allergens.

d. Implement Pollen Avoidance Techniques: On high, pollen days, try to stay indoors, especially during peak pollen times. Keep windows closed and use air conditioning to filter and cool the air. When returning from outdoor activities, rinse off and change clothes to remove pollen from your body and prevent it from spreading indoors.

e. Manage Pet Allergens: If you have allergies to pet dander, consider designating certain

Chapter Twelve

Sinusitis in Children

Sinusitis in Children: Navigating the Challenges and Promoting Healthy Sinuses

Sinusitis, the inflammation or infection of the sinuses, can affect people of all ages, including children. In fact, sinusitis is a common condition among children, and it poses unique challenges due to their developing immune systems and anatomical differences. Understanding sinusitis in children is essential for prompt diagnosis, appropriate treatment, and long, term sinus health. Below we will explore the characteristics of sinusitis in children, factors that contribute to its development, and strategies for prevention and management.

Understanding Sinusitis in Children: Sinusitis in children is similar to sinusitis in adults, involving the inflammation or infection of the sinuses. The sinuses are air, filled spaces located behind the forehead, cheeks, and eyes. In children, sinusitis can occur as acute or chronic, with similar symptoms but varying durations.

Factors Contributing to Sinusitis in Children:

a. Viral Infections: Sinusitis often follows a viral upper respiratory infection, such as the common cold. These infections can cause nasal congestion, increased mucus production, and impaired sinus drainage, leading to the development of sinusitis.

b. Allergies: Children with allergies are more prone to sinusitis. Allergic reactions can cause nasal inflammation and increased mucus production, creating an environment conducive to sinus infection.

c. Anatomical Factors: Children may have anatomical differences that increase their susceptibility to sinusitis. These include narrow sinus passages, nasal polyps, or a deviated nasal septum. These structural variations can hinder proper sinus drainage and increase the risk of infection.

d. Exposure to Irritants: Environmental factors such as exposure to tobacco smoke, pollutants, and allergens can contribute to the development of sinusitis in children. Irritants can trigger nasal inflammation and impair sinus function.

Recognizing Symptoms in Children:

a. Nasal Congestion: Children with sinusitis often experience nasal congestion or stuffiness. They may have difficulty breathing through the nose and may exhibit a nasal voice or snoring during sleep.

b. Discolored Nasal Discharge: Sinusitis can cause thick, yellow or green nasal discharge. Parents should monitor the color and consistency of their child's nasal discharge as a potential indicator of sinus infection.

c. Facial Pain and Pressure: Older children may complain of facial pain or pressure, particularly around the forehead, cheeks, or eyes. They may also experience headaches.

d. Coughing and Sore Throat: Sinus drainage can trigger coughing and a sore throat, especially when the mucus drips down the back of the throat.

e. Fatigue and Irritability: Young children with sinusitis may exhibit general fatigue, irritability, and difficulty sleeping. These symptoms can be attributed to the discomfort caused by nasal congestion and disrupted sleep patterns.

Preventive Measures for Sinusitis in Children:

a. Maintain Good Hygiene: Teach children proper hand hygiene, including regular handwashing with soap and water. This reduces the spread of germs and lowers the risk of respiratory infections that can lead to sinusitis.

b. Allergen Management: Identify and manage any allergies your child may have. Minimize exposure to allergens by regularly cleaning the home, using allergen, proof covers on pillows and mattresses, and avoiding known triggers.

c. Avoid Tobacco Smoke: Keep children away from tobacco smoke, as it can irritate the nasal passages and increase the risk of sinusitis. If you smoke, do so outside and away from your child.

d. Healthy Diet and Hydration: Encourage a balanced diet rich in fruits, vegetables, and whole grains.

Causes and Symptoms

Causes and Symptoms: Unraveling the Factors Behind Sinusitis

Sinusitis, a common condition affecting millions of people worldwide, is characterized by inflammation or infection of the sinuses. It can cause significant discomfort and disrupt daily life. Understanding the causes and recognizing the symptoms of sinusitis is crucial for prompt diagnosis, effective treatment, and prevention of complications. Below we will explore the various causes and symptoms of sinusitis, shedding light on the factors that contribute to its development and the signs that indicate its presence.

Understanding Sinusitis: Sinusitis occurs when the sinuses, which are air, filled cavities located around the nasal passages, become inflamed or infected. The sinuses play a crucial role in producing mucus, filtering air, and helping with voice resonance. When the sinuses are affected, it can lead to a range of symptoms and discomfort.

Causes of Sinusitis:

a. Viral Infections: The most common cause of sinusitis is a viral infection, such as the common cold or influenza. These infections can cause inflammation of the nasal passages and impair proper sinus drainage, leading to the development of sinusitis.

b. Bacterial Infections: In some cases, sinusitis may be caused by a bacterial infection. Bacteria can invade the sinuses when the nasal passages are inflamed or blocked, leading to the growth of bacteria and subsequent infection.

c. Allergies: Allergic reactions to environmental triggers, such as pollen, dust mites, or pet dander, can cause nasal inflammation and increased mucus production. This can obstruct the sinuses and contribute to the development of sinusitis.

d. Structural Abnormalities: Structural abnormalities within the nasal passages, such as a deviated nasal septum or nasal polyps, can obstruct proper sinus drainage and increase the risk of sinusitis.

e. Dental Infections: In some cases, dental infections, such as infected teeth or gum disease, can spread to the sinuses and lead to sinusitis. This occurs when the infection travels through the maxillary sinuses, which are located near the upper back teeth.

f. Environmental Factors: Exposure to environmental irritants, such as tobacco smoke, pollutants, and chemicals, can irritate the nasal passages and contribute to sinus inflammation and infection.

Common Symptoms of Sinusitis:

a. Nasal Congestion: One of the hallmark symptoms of sinusitis is nasal congestion or stuffiness. The nasal passages may feel blocked, making it difficult to breathe through the nose.

b. Discolored Nasal Discharge: Sinusitis can cause thick, discolored nasal discharge. The discharge may be yellow, green, or brown in color, indicating the presence of infection.

c. Facial Pain and Pressure: Sinusitis often leads to facial pain and pressure. This discomfort is typically felt in the forehead, cheeks, or around the eyes. The pain may worsen when bending forward or lying down.

d. Headaches: Sinus headaches are common in individuals with sinusitis. The pain is typically localized in the front of the head or around the eyes.

e. Loss of Smell and Taste: Sinusitis can affect the sense of smell and taste. Many individuals report a decreased ability to detect odors and a reduced enjoyment of food.

f. Coughing and Postnasal Drip: Sinus drainage can trigger a persistent cough or a sensation of mucus dripping down the back of the throat. This is known as postnasal drip.

Treatment and Prevention

Treatment and Prevention: Navigating the Path to Sinusitis Relief and Long, term Wellness

Sinusitis, the inflammation or infection of the sinuses, can cause significant discomfort and disrupt daily life. Fortunately, there are various treatment options available to alleviate symptoms and promote healing. Additionally, implementing preventive measures can help reduce the risk of sinusitis and maintain long, term sinus health. Below we will explore the treatment modalities for sinusitis and delve into effective prevention strategies to minimize its occurrence.

Treatment Options for Sinusitis:

Medications:

a. Nasal Decongestants: These medications help alleviate nasal congestion by shrinking swollen blood vessels in the nasal passages. They are available as over, the, counter sprays or oral formulations. However, nasal decongestant sprays should be used sparingly and for a limited duration to prevent rebound congestion.

b. Saline Nasal Irrigation: Saline solution rinses can help flush out mucus and allergens from the nasal passages, promoting sinus drainage and relieving symptoms. Neti pots or squeeze bottles are commonly used for nasal irrigation.

c. Nasal Steroid Sprays: These sprays reduce inflammation in the nasal passages and help alleviate symptoms such as nasal congestion, postnasal drip, and facial pain. They are available both over, the, counter and by prescription.

d. Antibiotics: If a bacterial infection is present or suspected, antibiotics may be prescribed to eliminate the infection. However, antibiotics are not routinely prescribed for all cases of sinusitis, as the majority of sinusitis cases are viral in nature.

e. Pain Relievers: Over, the, counter pain relievers such as acetaminophen or nonsteroidal anti, inflammatory drugs (NSAIDs) can help reduce facial pain, headaches, and fever associated with sinusitis.

Home Remedies and Self, care:

a. Warm Compresses: Applying warm compresses to the face can help relieve facial pain and pressure associated with sinusitis. The warmth promotes blood circulation and eases inflammation.

b. Steam Inhalation: Inhaling steam from a bowl of hot water or using a humidifier can help moisturize the nasal passages, promote sinus drainage, and alleviate congestion. Adding a few drops of essential oils, such as eucalyptus or peppermint, can provide additional relief.

c. Hydration: Drinking plenty of fluids helps thin mucus secretions, making it easier for the sinuses to drain. Opt for water, herbal teas, and clear broths to stay hydrated.

d. Rest and Sleep: Adequate rest and sleep allow the body to heal and recover. Make sure to prioritize quality sleep to support the immune system and promote overall well, being.

e. Nasal Irrigation: Regular use of saline nasal sprays or irrigation kits can help maintain clear nasal passages, reduce inflammation, and flush out irritants.

f. Avoiding Allergens and Irritants: Identify and avoid allergens that trigger sinusitis symptoms. Additionally, minimize exposure to irritants such as tobacco smoke, strong chemicals, and pollutants, which can exacerbate sinus inflammation.

Preventive Strategies for Sinusitis:

Allergy Management:

a. Identify Allergens: Determine the specific allergens that trigger sinusitis symptoms and take steps to minimize exposure. This may involve allergen testing or keeping a journal of symptoms to identify patterns.

b. Environmental Controls: Implement strategies to reduce allergens in the environment. Use air purifiers with HEPA filters, keep windows closed during high pollen seasons, and regularly clean bedding to minimize dust mites and pet dander.

When to See a Doctor

When to See a Doctor: Decoding the Signals of Sinusitis

Sinusitis, the inflammation or infection of the sinuses, can cause significant discomfort and disrupt daily life. While many cases of sinusitis can be managed at home with self, care measures and over, the, counter medications, there are instances when it is necessary to seek medical attention. Recognizing the signs and knowing when to consult a doctor is crucial for proper diagnosis, appropriate treatment, and prevention of complications. Below we will explore the red flags and indicators that warrant a visit to the doctor when dealing with sinusitis.

Persistent or Worsening Symptoms:

a. Duration of Symptoms: Most cases of acute sinusitis resolve within 7, 10 days with proper self, care. However, if symptoms persist beyond this timeframe or worsen over time, it is advisable to seek medical evaluation.

b. Intensity of Symptoms: Severe or debilitating symptoms such as intense facial pain, high fever, or severe headache should not be ignored. These may indicate a more severe infection or other underlying issues requiring medical attention.

Recurrent Sinusitis:

a. Frequent Episodes: If you experience recurring episodes of sinusitis, with symptoms occurring multiple times throughout the year, it is recommended to consult a doctor. This may indicate an underlying issue that needs to be addressed, such as chronic sinusitis or structural abnormalities.

b. Failed Self, Care Measures: If your symptoms persist despite diligent self, care efforts, including rest, hydration, and appropriate over, the, counter treatments, it is advisable to seek medical advice.

Severe or Unusual Symptoms:

a. High Fever: A persistent high fever, typically above 102°F (38.9°C), may indicate a more severe infection or complication that requires medical attention.

b. Severe Facial Pain: Intense facial pain that is not alleviated by over, the, counter pain relievers may indicate a more severe infection or the presence of complications such as a sinus abscess.

c. Vision Problems: If you experience sudden vision changes, double vision, or eye, related symptoms such as swelling, redness, or bulging, it is important to seek immediate medical attention, as these may indicate severe complications.

d. Neurological Symptoms: Neurological symptoms such as confusion, seizures, or severe headaches accompanied by neck stiffness should not be ignored. These symptoms may be signs of severe infection or other underlying conditions that require urgent medical evaluation.

Concerns in Specific Populations:

a. Children: If your child is experiencing symptoms of sinusitis, it is advisable to consult a pediatrician. Children may exhibit different symptoms than adults, and their developing immune systems require special attention.

b. Elderly Individuals: Elderly individuals may be more susceptible to severe infections and complications. If an elderly person experiences sinusitis symptoms, it is important to seek medical evaluation promptly.

Underlying Health Conditions:

a. Immune, compromised Individuals: If you have a weakened immune system due to conditions such as HIV/AIDS, chemotherapy, or organ transplantation, it is important to seek medical attention at the first sign of sinusitis. These individuals are at a higher risk of developing severe infections and complications.

b. Chronic Health Conditions: If you have underlying chronic health conditions, such as asthma, cystic fibrosis, or nasal polyps, it is advisable to consult a doctor for proper management of sinusitis to prevent complications and ensure effective treatment.

Occupational or Environmental Factors:

a. Occupational Exposures: If you work in an environment with high exposure to allergens, pollutants, or irritants, such as construction sites or factories, and you develop sinusitis symptoms, it is recommended to seek medical advice.

Chapter Thirteen

Sinusitis and Other Health Conditions

Sinusitis and Other Health Conditions: Unveiling the Connections and Coexisting Challenges

Sinusitis, the inflammation or infection of the sinuses, can be influenced by and coexist with various other health conditions. Understanding the relationships between sinusitis and these conditions is crucial for comprehensive management and improved overall well, being. Below we will explore the connections between sinusitis and other health conditions, shedding light on how they can influence each other and the challenges they present.

Allergies:

a. Allergic Rhinitis: Allergic rhinitis, commonly known as hay fever, is an allergic reaction to environmental triggers such as pollen, dust mites, or pet dander. Allergic rhinitis and sinusitis often coexist, as the inflammation and increased mucus production in allergic rhinitis can obstruct the sinuses and lead to sinusitis.

b. Impact: Allergic rhinitis can exacerbate sinusitis symptoms and make them more difficult to manage. Effective management of allergic rhinitis, including allergen avoidance and appropriate medication, can help minimize the occurrence and severity of sinusitis.

Asthma:

a. Coexistence: There is a significant association between sinusitis and asthma. The two conditions often coexist, and individuals with both conditions may experience more severe symptoms and complications.

b. Shared Inflammation: Both sinusitis and asthma involve inflammation of the airways. Inflammation in the sinuses can trigger or worsen asthma symptoms, and vice versa. Addressing sinusitis can help improve asthma control and vice versa.

c. Management: Managing both conditions concurrently is essential for optimal symptom control and improved quality of life. This may involve medication management, allergen avoidance, and regular monitoring by healthcare professionals.

Nasal Polyps:

a. Relationship: Nasal polyps are noncancerous growths that develop in the lining of the nasal passages or sinuses. They can contribute to the development of sinusitis by obstructing sinus drainage and promoting the growth of bacteria or fungi.

b. Impact: The presence of nasal polyps can make sinusitis symptoms more persistent and difficult to treat. Effective management of nasal polyps, including medication and, in some cases, surgical intervention, can help alleviate sinusitis symptoms and improve sinus health.

Cystic Fibrosis:

a. Impact: Cystic fibrosis (CF) is a genetic disorder that affects multiple organs, including the respiratory system. Individuals with CF are at a higher risk of developing sinusitis due to the thickening of mucus in the airways, which impairs proper sinus drainage.

b. Chronic Sinusitis: Sinusitis in individuals with CF is often chronic and recurrent. Effective management of CF, including airway clearance techniques and regular use of prescribed medications, is crucial in preventing and managing sinusitis.

Immunodeficiency Disorders:

a. Impact: Immunodeficiency disorders, such as primary immunodeficiency or acquired immunodeficiency syndrome (AIDS), can weaken the immune system's ability to fight off infections, making individuals more susceptible to sinusitis.

b. Recurrent Infections: Sinusitis in individuals with immunodeficiency disorders may be recurrent and more challenging to treat. Close monitoring and appropriate management of the underlying immunodeficiency disorder, along with targeted treatment for sinusitis, are essential.

Gastroesophageal Reflux Disease (GERD):

a. Relationship: There is a growing recognition of the link between sinusitis and GERD, a condition characterized by the reflux of stomach acid into the esophagus. It is believed that the refluxed acid can reach the back of the throat and enter the sinuses, leading to inflammation and sinusitis.

Asthma and Sinusitis

Asthma and Sinusitis: Unraveling the Connections for Comprehensive Care

Asthma and sinusitis are two distinct respiratory conditions that often coexist and can influence each other's severity and management. Understanding the relationship between asthma and sinusitis is essential for comprehensive care and improved quality of life for individuals dealing with both conditions. Below we will explore the connections between asthma and sinusitis, shedding light on how they can interact and the challenges they present.

Coexistence of Asthma and Sinusitis:

a. Shared Airways: Asthma and sinusitis share a common link through the respiratory system. Both conditions involve inflammation of the airways, although they occur in different parts of the respiratory tract. The inflammation in one area can influence the other, leading to shared symptoms and exacerbations.

b. Impact on Asthma: Sinusitis can worsen asthma symptoms and trigger asthma attacks. Inflammation in the sinuses can lead to increased mucus production, postnasal drip, and nasal congestion, which can aggravate asthma symptoms such as coughing, wheezing, and shortness of breath.

c. Impact on Sinusitis: Similarly, asthma, related inflammation can affect the sinuses. The airway inflammation in asthma can obstruct proper sinus drainage, leading to an increased risk of sinusitis. Additionally, the use of asthma medications, such as inhaled corticosteroids, can increase the susceptibility to sinusitis.

Common Factors Contributing to Asthma and Sinusitis:

a. Allergies: Allergies play a significant role in both asthma and sinusitis. Allergic reactions to environmental triggers such as pollen, dust mites, or pet dander can cause inflammation in the nasal passages and sinuses, leading to symptoms of sinusitis and triggering asthma attacks.

b. Inflammation: Inflammation is a hallmark feature of both asthma and sinusitis. Chronic inflammation in the airways can affect both the lungs and the sinuses, leading to persistent symptoms in both conditions.

c. Immune System Response: The immune system plays a crucial role in both asthma and sinusitis. An overactive or dysfunctional immune response can contribute to the development and progression of both conditions.

Challenges in Diagnosis:

a. Overlapping Symptoms: Asthma and sinusitis share some common symptoms, such as coughing, wheezing, and nasal congestion. This overlap can make it challenging to differentiate between the two conditions, leading to delayed or incorrect diagnosis.

b. Misinterpretation of Symptoms: Sinusitis symptoms, such as facial pain or headache, may be mistakenly attributed to asthma, related symptoms, resulting in inadequate treatment for sinusitis.

Impact on Treatment and Management:

a. Medication Considerations: The treatment and management of asthma and sinusitis often require a multifaceted approach. Medications used for asthma, such as inhaled corticosteroids, can also help manage the airway inflammation associated with sinusitis. However, additional medications specific to sinusitis may be required, such as nasal corticosteroids or saline rinses.

b. Treatment Integration: Coordinating treatment between healthcare providers specializing in asthma and sinusitis is important to ensure a comprehensive approach to care. This may involve collaboration between pulmonologists, allergists, and otolaryngologists (ear, nose, and throat specialists).

c. Allergy Management: Addressing underlying allergies is crucial for managing both asthma and sinusitis. Identifying and avoiding allergens, undergoing allergy testing, and considering allergen immunotherapy (allergy shots) can help reduce the frequency and severity of symptoms in both conditions.

Sinusitis and Sleep Apnea

Sinusitis and Sleep Apnea: Unraveling the Complex Relationship

Sinusitis and sleep apnea are two distinct conditions that can coexist and influence each other in various ways. Understanding the relationship between sinusitis and sleep apnea is essential for comprehensive management and improved quality of life for individuals dealing with both conditions. Below we will explore the complex connections between sinusitis and sleep apnea, shedding light on how they can interact and the challenges they present.

Coexistence of Sinusitis and Sleep Apnea:

a. Impact of Sinusitis on Sleep Apnea: Sinusitis, the inflammation or infection of the sinuses, can worsen sleep apnea symptoms. Nasal congestion, postnasal drip, and inflammation in the airways due to sinusitis can obstruct the airflow, exacerbating the breathing difficulties associated with sleep apnea. This can lead to more frequent episodes of interrupted breathing during sleep.

b. Impact of Sleep Apnea on Sinusitis: Sleep apnea, characterized by repeated pauses in breathing during sleep, can contribute to the development or worsening of sinusitis. The abnormal breathing patterns in sleep apnea can cause dryness in the nasal passages, impair nasal clearance, and promote bacterial growth, leading to sinusitis.

Shared Risk Factors:

a. Nasal Anatomy: Anatomical abnormalities, such as a deviated septum or nasal polyps, can contribute to both sinusitis and sleep apnea. These structural issues can obstruct the nasal passages, leading to chronic inflammation, nasal congestion, and impaired breathing during sleep.

b. Allergies: Allergies play a significant role in both sinusitis and sleep apnea. Allergic reactions to environmental triggers can cause nasal congestion, inflammation, and increased mucus production, exacerbating symptoms in both conditions.

c. Obesity: Obesity is a common risk factor for both sinusitis and sleep apnea. Excess weight can contribute to chronic inflammation, compromise nasal airflow, and increase the likelihood of developing sleep apnea and sinusitis.

Challenges in Diagnosis:

a. Overlapping Symptoms: Sinusitis and sleep apnea share some common symptoms, such as nasal congestion, snoring, and fatigue. This overlap can make it challenging to differentiate between the two conditions, leading to delayed or incorrect diagnosis.

b. Misinterpretation of Symptoms: Symptoms of sinusitis, such as facial pain or headache, may be mistakenly attributed to sleep apnea, related symptoms, resulting in inadequate treatment for sinusitis.

Impact on Treatment and Management:

a. Sinusitis Treatment and Sleep Apnea: Effectively managing sinusitis can help improve sleep apnea symptoms. Treating the underlying sinus inflammation, such as through nasal corticosteroids or saline rinses, can alleviate nasal congestion, improve nasal airflow, and reduce sleep apnea symptoms.

b. Sleep Apnea Treatment and Sinusitis: Managing sleep apnea can also have a positive impact on sinusitis symptoms. Continuous positive airway pressure (CPAP) therapy, a common treatment for sleep apnea, can help maintain open airways and improve nasal airflow, reducing the risk of sinusitis.

c. Coordinated Care: Coordinating treatment between healthcare providers specializing in sinusitis and sleep apnea is crucial for comprehensive management. Collaboration between otolaryngologists (ear, nose, and throat specialists) and sleep medicine specialists can ensure a holistic approach to care.

d. Addressing Shared Risk Factors: Managing shared risk factors, such as allergies or obesity, can play a significant role in improving both sinusitis and sleep apnea. Addressing allergies through allergen avoidance or immunotherapy and implementing lifestyle changes for weight loss can have a positive impact on both conditions.

Sinusitis and Migraines

Sinusitis and Migraines: Unraveling the Intricate Connection

Sinusitis and migraines are two distinct conditions that can share common symptoms and often coexist. Understanding the relationship between sinusitis and migraines is crucial for proper diagnosis, effective treatment, and improved quality of life for individuals dealing with both conditions. Below we will explore the intricate connection between sinusitis and migraines, shedding light on how they can interact and the challenges they present.

Overlapping Symptoms:

a. Facial Pain: Both sinusitis and migraines can cause facial pain, making it difficult to differentiate between the two conditions. Sinusitis, related facial pain often manifests as pressure or aching in the cheeks, forehead, or around the eyes, whereas migraines are typically characterized by throbbing or pulsating pain on one side of the head.

b. Headache: Headaches are a common symptom in both sinusitis and migraines. Sinusitis, related headaches are often described as a dull ache, whereas migraines are intense, often accompanied by nausea, sensitivity to light and sound, and worsened by physical activity.

c. Nasal Symptoms: Nasal congestion, postnasal drip, and sinus pressure are common in both sinusitis and migraines. In sinusitis, these symptoms are caused by inflammation and blockage of the sinuses, whereas in migraines, they can occur as part of the neurological cascade associated with migraines.

Sinusitis Triggering Migraines:

a. Inflammation: The inflammation caused by sinusitis can trigger migraines in susceptible individuals. The release of inflammatory mediators during sinusitis can activate pain pathways and lead to the onset of migraines.

b. Nasal Congestion: Nasal congestion associated with sinusitis can contribute to the development of migraines. The increased pressure in the sinuses can impact blood flow and trigger migraines in individuals who are prone to them.

Migraines Triggering Sinusitis:

a. Vascular Changes: Migraines can cause changes in blood flow to the sinuses, leading to nasal congestion and inflammation. This can increase the risk of developing sinusitis during migraine episodes.

b. Altered Immune Response: Migraines may influence the immune response in the sinuses, making individuals more susceptible to sinus infections. Changes in immune function during migraines can impair the body's ability to fight off bacterial or viral pathogens, contributing to sinusitis.

Challenges in Diagnosis:

a. Symptom Overlap: The overlapping symptoms of sinusitis and migraines can make it challenging to accurately diagnose the underlying condition. Misdiagnosis or delayed diagnosis may lead to ineffective or inappropriate treatments.

b. Coexistence: It is possible for individuals to have both sinusitis and migraines simultaneously, further complicating the diagnostic process. Careful evaluation by a healthcare professional is essential to differentiate between the two conditions and develop an appropriate treatment plan.

Impact on Treatment and Management:

a. Sinusitis Treatment and Migraines: Effectively managing sinusitis can help alleviate migraine symptoms in individuals who experience migraines as a result of sinusitis triggers. Treating sinusitis, related inflammation, nasal congestion, and infection can reduce the frequency and intensity of migraines.

b. Migraine Treatment and Sinusitis: Addressing migraines through appropriate medication and lifestyle management can help reduce the risk of developing sinusitis. Migraine, specific medications, such as triptans or preventive medications, can be used to manage migraines and potentially reduce sinusitis exacerbations.

c. Coordinated Care: Coordinating care between healthcare providers specializing in sinusitis and migraine management is crucial for a comprehensive approach.

Chapter Fourteen

Mental Health and Sinusitis

Mental Health and Sinusitis: Exploring the Mind, Body Connection

Sinusitis, the inflammation or infection of the sinuses, can have a profound impact on mental health and overall well, being. The interplay between sinusitis and mental health is complex, with each influencing the other in various ways. Below we will delve into the fascinating relationship between mental health and sinusitis, shedding light on the connections and challenges that arise.

Impact of Sinusitis on Mental Health:

a. Physical Discomfort: Sinusitis can cause significant physical discomfort, including facial pain, headaches, nasal congestion, and fatigue. The chronic nature of sinusitis, with recurrent or persistent symptoms, can take a toll on an individual's mental well, being, leading to frustration, irritability, and reduced quality of life.

b. Sleep Disturbances: Sinusitis, related symptoms, such as nasal congestion and postnasal drip, can disrupt sleep patterns, resulting in poor sleep quality or sleep deprivation. Sleep disturbances can contribute to mood disturbances, fatigue, and reduced cognitive function, impacting overall mental health.

c. Impact on Daily Functioning: Chronic sinusitis can affect daily activities and productivity. Constant discomfort, reduced energy levels, and impaired concentration can hinder one's ability to perform tasks effectively, leading to increased stress, anxiety, and feelings of overwhelm.

d. Psychological Impact: The persistent nature of sinusitis and its impact on physical and social functioning can contribute to psychological distress. Individuals may experience increased levels of anxiety, depression, and a diminished sense of well, being.

Mental Health Factors Influencing Sinusitis:

a. Stress: Chronic stress can weaken the immune system and make individuals more susceptible to infections, including sinusitis. Additionally, stress can exacerbate sinusitis symptoms and prolong recovery.

b. Emotional Factors: Emotional factors, such as anxiety and depression, can affect the immune response and increase susceptibility to infections. Emotional distress may also impact self, care practices, making individuals less likely to manage sinusitis effectively.

Challenges in Diagnosis and Treatment:

a. Diagnostic Difficulties: The symptoms of sinusitis and mental health conditions can overlap, leading to diagnostic challenges. Symptoms such as fatigue, headaches, and cognitive difficulties can be attributed to both sinusitis and mental health disorders. Accurate diagnosis requires a comprehensive evaluation by healthcare professionals.

b. Treatment Compliance: Mental health conditions can affect treatment adherence and motivation to manage sinusitis effectively. Individuals experiencing mental health challenges may find it difficult to follow treatment plans, leading to suboptimal outcomes in sinusitis management.

Integrated Management Approach:

a. Addressing Physical and Mental Health: A holistic approach that considers both physical and mental health is crucial in managing sinusitis. Treating sinusitis effectively can help alleviate physical symptoms and improve overall well, being, positively impacting mental health.

b. Psychological Support: Providing psychological support is important in addressing the emotional impact of sinusitis. Counseling or therapy can help individuals develop coping strategies, manage stress, and improve their mental resilience in the face of chronic illness.

c. Stress Management Techniques: Implementing stress management techniques, such as mindfulness meditation, relaxation exercises, and lifestyle modifications, can help individuals reduce stress levels, enhance immune function, and potentially minimize the risk of sinusitis.

d. Collaborative Care: Collaborative care between healthcare professionals specializing in sinusitis and mental health is beneficial in providing integrated and comprehensive management. Close communication and coordination can ensure that both physical and mental health needs are addressed effectively.

Self, Care Practices:

a. Lifestyle Modifications: Adopting a healthy lifestyle can support both physical and mental well, being.

Impact on Quality of Life

The Impact of Sinusitis on Quality of Life: Navigating the Challenges

Sinusitis, the inflammation or infection of the sinuses, can have a significant impact on an individual's quality of life. The physical discomfort, persistent symptoms, and limitations it imposes can affect various aspects of daily living. Understanding the implications of sinusitis on quality of life is crucial for comprehensive management and improving overall well, being. Below we will explore the multifaceted impact of sinusitis on quality of life and the challenges it presents.

Physical Discomfort:

a. Facial Pain and Headaches: Sinusitis often causes facial pain, pressure, and headaches. These symptoms can be debilitating and impact one's ability to concentrate, work, and engage in daily activities. The constant discomfort can lead to frustration, irritability, and reduced enjoyment of life.

b. Nasal Congestion and Breathing Difficulties: Chronic nasal congestion and difficulty breathing can significantly impact quality of life. Restricted airflow can affect sleep, energy levels, and physical activities, leading to fatigue and decreased participation in social and recreational activities.

c. Fatigue and Reduced Energy: The persistent nature of sinusitis and the associated symptoms can result in fatigue and reduced energy levels. This can affect productivity, social interactions, and engagement in hobbies and interests.

Impact on Daily Activities:

a. Work and Productivity: Sinusitis can interfere with work productivity due to symptoms such as pain, fatigue, and difficulty concentrating. Frequent absences or decreased performance can affect job satisfaction and professional growth.

b. Social Interactions: Sinusitis can limit social interactions and engagement in social activities. The physical discomfort, fatigue, and concern over symptoms may lead individuals to withdraw from social gatherings, impacting relationships and overall well, being.

c. Emotional Well, being: Chronic sinusitis can lead to emotional distress, including frustration, irritability, and sadness. Dealing with persistent symptoms and their impact on daily life can contribute to feelings of helplessness and reduced overall emotional well, being.

Sleep Disturbances:

a. Disrupted Sleep Patterns: Nasal congestion, postnasal drip, and pain can disrupt sleep patterns in individuals with sinusitis. Sleep disturbances can lead to poor sleep quality, daytime fatigue, and impaired cognitive function, further impacting quality of life.

b. Impact on Mood: Lack of quality sleep can contribute to mood disturbances, including increased irritability, anxiety, and depression. The cycle of poor sleep and negative emotions can further exacerbate the impact of sinusitis on overall well, being.

Psychological and Emotional Impact:

a. Emotional Distress: The chronic nature of sinusitis and the associated symptoms can cause emotional distress. Individuals may experience frustration, anxiety, and depression as they navigate the challenges of living with a chronic condition.

b. Self, esteem and Body Image: Visible symptoms such as facial swelling, nasal discharge, or redness can impact self, esteem and body image. Concerns about appearance may lead to self, consciousness and avoidance of social situations.

c. Limitations on Activities: Sinusitis can impose limitations on physical activities, hobbies, and interests. Individuals may feel restricted in their ability to participate in sports, exercise, or other recreational activities, which can impact self, identity and overall satisfaction with life.

Challenges in Treatment and Management:

a. Misdiagnosis or Delayed Diagnosis: Sinusitis can be challenging to diagnose accurately, leading to delayed or ineffective treatment. This can prolong symptoms and their impact on quality of life.

b. Treatment Side Effects: Some sinusitis treatments, such as nasal corticosteroids or antibiotics, may have side effects that can further impact daily functioning and well, being.

Coping with Chronic Sinusitis

Coping with Chronic Sinusitis: Navigating the Challenges with Resilience

Chronic sinusitis, a condition characterized by long, lasting inflammation or infection of the sinuses, can significantly impact an individual's physical and emotional well, being. The persistent nature of the symptoms, the challenges in finding effective treatment, and the impact on daily life can be overwhelming. However, with the right strategies and support, individuals can learn to cope with chronic sinusitis and maintain a good quality of life. Below we will explore various coping mechanisms and strategies to help individuals navigate the challenges of living with chronic sinusitis.

Education and Self, Advocacy:

a. Understanding the Condition: Educating oneself about chronic sinusitis is essential in managing the condition effectively. Learning about the causes, symptoms, treatment options, and lifestyle modifications can empower individuals to make informed decisions about their healthcare.

b. Seeking Knowledgeable Healthcare Providers: Finding healthcare providers who specialize in sinusitis and have experience with chronic cases can make a significant difference. Building a strong healthcare team and establishing open communication can ensure that individuals receive appropriate treatment and support.

c. Self, Advocacy: Being an active participant in one's healthcare journey is crucial. Individuals should communicate their symptoms, concerns, and treatment preferences to their healthcare providers. Asking questions, seeking second opinions when necessary, and actively engaging in treatment decisions can help individuals feel more empowered and in control.

Lifestyle Modifications:

a. Nasal Hygiene: Practicing good nasal hygiene can help alleviate symptoms and prevent complications. This includes regularly rinsing the nasal passages with saline solutions, using humidifiers to keep the air moist, and avoiding environmental triggers such as irritants and allergens.

b. Healthy Diet and Exercise: Maintaining a healthy lifestyle can support overall well, being and immune function. Consuming a balanced diet rich in fruits, vegetables, and whole grains, along with regular exercise, can boost the body's defenses and potentially reduce the frequency and severity of sinusitis symptoms.

c. Stress Management: Stress can exacerbate sinusitis symptoms and impact overall well, being. Implementing stress management techniques such as meditation, deep breathing exercises, yoga, or engaging in hobbies and activities that promote relaxation can help individuals better cope with the challenges of chronic sinusitis.

Symptom Management:

a. Medication Adherence: Following prescribed medication regimens and adhering to treatment plans is crucial for managing chronic sinusitis. This includes taking prescribed antibiotics, nasal corticosteroids, or antihistamines as directed and completing the full course of treatment.

b. Pain Management: Chronic sinusitis can cause facial pain and headaches. Over, the, counter pain relievers or prescribed medications can help alleviate discomfort. However, it is important to consult with a healthcare provider before taking any medications, especially if there are pre, existing medical conditions or interactions with other medications.

c. Nasal Irrigation: Regular nasal irrigation using saline solutions can help clear mucus, reduce inflammation, and alleviate congestion. Neti pots, squeeze bottles, or nasal sprays can be used to deliver the saline solution to the nasal passages.

Emotional Support:

a. Seek Emotional Support: Living with chronic sinusitis can be emotionally challenging. Seeking support from friends, family, or support groups can provide a safe space to share experiences, gain insights, and receive emotional validation.

b. Counseling or Therapy: Individual or group therapy can help individuals develop coping strategies, manage stress, and address the emotional impact of living with a chronic condition. A trained therapist can provide guidance and support in navigating the emotional challenges associated with chronic sinusitis.

Seeking Support

Seeking Support: The Importance of Community in Dealing with Sinusitis

Living with sinusitis can be challenging, both physically and emotionally. The chronic nature of the condition, along with its associated symptoms and impact on daily life, can leave individuals feeling overwhelmed and isolated. However, seeking support from others can make a significant difference in managing sinusitis effectively and improving overall well, being. Below we will explore the importance of seeking support and the various avenues available to individuals dealing with sinusitis.

Understanding the Benefits of Support:

a. Emotional Validation: Connecting with others who are experiencing similar challenges can provide a sense of validation and understanding. Sharing experiences, frustrations, and triumphs with individuals who can relate can help alleviate feelings of isolation and offer a sense of belonging.

b. Knowledge and Resources: Engaging with a supportive community can provide access to a wealth of knowledge and resources. Others' experiences and insights can offer practical tips, coping strategies, and information on treatment options that individuals may not have considered.

c. Emotional Well, being: Social support can have a positive impact on emotional well, being. It can reduce stress levels, enhance mood, and provide a sense of comfort during difficult times. Knowing that one is not alone in their struggles can foster resilience and emotional strength.

Support from Friends and Family:

a. Open Communication: Establishing open and honest communication with friends and family members is vital. Sharing experiences, concerns, and needs can help loved ones better understand the challenges faced by individuals with sinusitis and provide the necessary support.

b. Practical Assistance: Friends and family can offer practical help, such as accompanying individuals to medical appointments, assisting with household chores, or providing transportation when needed. Their support can ease the burden of managing sinusitis and allow individuals to focus on their well, being.

c. Emotional Support: Loved ones can provide a listening ear and offer emotional support during challenging times. Simply having someone to talk to, share fears and frustrations, and receive empathy can be immensely beneficial for individuals dealing with sinusitis.

Online Communities and Support Groups:

a. Virtual Support Networks: Online communities and support groups provide a platform for individuals to connect, share experiences, and exchange information about living with sinusitis. These platforms offer a sense of community and can be accessed from the comfort of one's home.

b. Access to Information: Online support groups often provide valuable resources, including articles, research updates, and treatment options. These resources can help individuals stay informed and make informed decisions about their healthcare.

c. Anonymous Support: Some individuals may prefer to seek support anonymously. Online communities allow individuals to share their experiences and concerns without disclosing personal information, providing a safe and non, judgmental space to express themselves.

Professional Support:

a. Healthcare Providers: Seeking support from healthcare professionals who specialize in sinusitis is crucial. These professionals can provide accurate diagnosis, recommend appropriate treatment options, and offer guidance on managing symptoms and improving quality of life.

b. Mental Health Professionals: Mental health professionals, such as therapists or counselors, can help individuals navigate the emotional impact of sinusitis. They can provide coping strategies, assist with stress management, and address any psychological distress associated with the condition.

c. Patient Advocacy Organizations: Patient advocacy organizations dedicated to sinusitis can offer a wealth of support and resources. They may provide educational materials, support hotlines, and connections to local support groups, giving individuals the opportunity to connect with others facing similar challenges.

Self, Help Strategies:

a. Journaling: Keeping a journal to document thoughts, emotions, and experiences can be therapeutic. It allows individuals to reflect on their journey, identify triggers or patterns, and track their progress.

Chapter Fifteen

The Role of Diet and Nutrition

The Role of Diet and Nutrition in Managing Sinusitis: Nourishing the Body for Relief

When it comes to managing sinusitis, a condition characterized by inflammation or infection of the sinuses, diet and nutrition play a crucial role. While they may not cure sinusitis, a healthy and balanced diet can support the immune system, reduce inflammation, and alleviate symptoms. Below we will explore the impact of diet and nutrition on sinusitis and discuss key dietary recommendations to manage the condition effectively.

The Anti, Inflammatory Diet:

Sinusitis involves inflammation of the sinus cavities, and adopting an anti, inflammatory diet can help reduce inflammation and ease symptoms. The following dietary principles are associated with an anti, inflammatory approach:

a. Increase Intake of Fruits and Vegetables: Fresh fruits and vegetables are rich in antioxidants, vitamins, minerals, and phytochemicals that have anti, inflammatory properties. Aim to include a variety of colorful fruits and vegetables in your daily meals.

b. Focus on Whole Grains: Whole grains such as quinoa, brown rice, and whole wheat bread provide essential nutrients and fiber. They help stabilize blood sugar levels and promote overall health, including reducing inflammation.

c. Incorporate Healthy Fats: Include sources of healthy fats in your diet, such as avocados, nuts, seeds, and olive oil. These fats contain omega, 3 fatty acids, which have anti, inflammatory properties.

d. Limit Processed Foods and Added Sugars: Processed foods and added sugars can contribute to inflammation and weaken the immune system. Minimize the consumption of processed snacks, sugary drinks, and foods high in trans fats.

Hydration:

Staying well, hydrated is essential for managing sinusitis. Proper hydration helps thin mucus secretions, promotes nasal drainage, and prevents dehydration, which can worsen symptoms. Consider the following tips:

a. Drink Plenty of Water: Aim to drink at least eight glasses of water per day to maintain adequate hydration. Additionally, warm fluids like herbal teas or clear broths can provide additional relief.

b. Use a Humidifier: Dry air can aggravate sinusitis symptoms. Using a humidifier can add moisture to the air and help keep nasal passages lubricated.

c. Limit Alcohol and Caffeine: Both alcohol and caffeine can contribute to dehydration. Limit your consumption of alcoholic and caffeinated beverages, as they may worsen sinusitis symptoms.

Nutrients and Supplements:

Certain nutrients and supplements have shown potential in supporting sinus health and reducing inflammation. However, it is important to consult with a healthcare provider before starting any new supplements. Some nutrients and supplements that may be beneficial include:

a. Vitamin C: Vitamin C supports immune function and has antioxidant properties. It can be found in citrus fruits, berries, kiwi, and leafy green vegetables.

b. Omega, 3 Fatty Acids: Omega, 3 fatty acids have anti, inflammatory effects. Good sources include fatty fish like salmon, trout, and sardines, as well as chia seeds, flaxseeds, and walnuts.

c. Probiotics: Probiotics promote a healthy gut microbiome and can support immune function. They can be found in fermented foods like yogurt, kefir, sauerkraut, and kimchi.

d. Quercetin: Quercetin is a flavonoid with anti, inflammatory properties. It can be found in foods such as onions, apples, berries, and green tea.

Potential Trigger Foods:

While there is no universal list of trigger foods for sinusitis, some individuals may find that certain foods worsen their symptoms.

Foods that May Help

Foods that May Help Alleviate Sinusitis: Nourishing Choices for Relief

When it comes to managing sinusitis, a condition characterized by inflammation or infection of the sinuses, certain foods can play a beneficial role. While no specific food can cure sinusitis, incorporating a variety of nutrient, rich foods into your diet can support your immune system, reduce inflammation, and alleviate symptoms. Below we will explore some foods that may help alleviate sinusitis symptoms and promote overall sinus health.

Citrus Fruits:

Citrus fruits such as oranges, lemons, grapefruits, and tangerines are rich in vitamin C, a powerful antioxidant that supports the immune system. Vitamin C helps strengthen the body's natural defenses and may help reduce the duration and severity of sinusitis symptoms. These fruits are also refreshing and can provide relief from congestion.

Berries:

Berries like strawberries, blueberries, raspberries, and blackberries are packed with antioxidants, vitamins, and minerals. They contain high levels of vitamin C, which can help boost the immune system and reduce inflammation. Berries also provide dietary fiber, which supports gut health and overall well, being.

Garlic and Onions:

Garlic and onions belong to the Allium family and contain compounds with antimicrobial and anti, inflammatory properties. These sulfur, containing vegetables have been traditionally used to support respiratory health. Adding them to your meals can enhance flavor while providing potential benefits for sinusitis management.

Ginger and Turmeric:

Ginger and turmeric are known for their anti, inflammatory properties. Ginger has long been used to alleviate respiratory conditions and may help reduce inflammation in the sinuses. Turmeric contains curcumin, a compound with potent anti, inflammatory effects. Adding ginger and turmeric to dishes or preparing warm beverages with them can be soothing and supportive for sinus health.

Leafy Greens:

Leafy greens such as spinach, kale, and Swiss chard are excellent sources of vitamins, minerals, and antioxidants. They provide essential nutrients like vitamin C, vitamin E, and beta, carotene, which support the immune system and combat inflammation. Incorporating leafy greens into your diet can contribute to overall sinus health and well, being.

Omega, 3 Fatty Acids:

Omega, 3 fatty acids have anti, inflammatory properties and may help reduce inflammation in the sinuses. Fatty fish like salmon, trout, and sardines are rich sources of omega, 3s. Consuming these fish two to three times a week can provide the necessary omega, 3 fatty acids to support sinus health. If you follow a vegetarian or vegan diet, plant, based sources of omega, 3s include chia seeds, flaxseeds, and walnuts.

Probiotic, Rich Foods:

Probiotics are beneficial bacteria that support a healthy gut microbiome and immune system. They can help regulate inflammation and promote overall well, being. Foods such as yogurt, kefir, sauerkraut, kimchi, and other fermented foods contain probiotics. Adding these foods to your diet can help support sinus health.

Spicy Foods:

Spicy foods like chili peppers, cayenne pepper, and horseradish contain compounds such as capsaicin, which can help relieve sinus congestion. These ingredients may temporarily open up nasal passages and promote sinus drainage, providing relief from symptoms.

Warm Broths and Soups:

Warm broths and soups, particularly those made from homemade bone broth or vegetable, based stocks, can provide nourishment and hydration.

The warmth and steam from soups can help relieve congestion, soothe the throat, and provide comfort during sinusitis episodes.

Foods to Avoid

Foods to Avoid for Sinusitis: Making Informed Dietary Choices for Relief

When it comes to managing sinusitis, a condition characterized by inflammation or infection of the sinuses, certain foods can potentially exacerbate symptoms or trigger allergic reactions. While individual sensitivities may vary, being mindful of the foods that can worsen sinusitis can help alleviate discomfort and promote overall sinus health. Below we will explore some common foods that may aggravate sinusitis symptoms and offer suggestions for making informed dietary choices.

Dairy Products:

Dairy products such as milk, cheese, and yogurt are known to cause increased mucus production in some individuals. This excess mucus can further congest the sinuses and worsen symptoms of sinusitis. If you notice that consuming dairy products leads to increased congestion or worsened sinus symptoms, it may be beneficial to reduce or avoid them.

Processed and Fried Foods:

Processed and fried foods tend to be high in unhealthy fats, sodium, and additives. These foods can promote inflammation in the body, including the sinuses. Additionally, the high sodium content in processed foods can contribute to water retention and worsen congestion. Opt for whole, unprocessed foods whenever possible.

Sugary Foods and Beverages:

Foods and beverages high in added sugars can contribute to inflammation and weaken the immune system. They can also disrupt the balance of beneficial bacteria in the gut, potentially affecting overall health and immune function. Avoid or limit the intake of sugary snacks, desserts, sweetened beverages, and processed foods.

Caffeine and Alcohol:

Both caffeine and alcohol can have dehydrating effects on the body, which can worsen sinusitis symptoms. Caffeine can also constrict blood vessels and lead to increased congestion. Limit your consumption of caffeinated beverages like coffee, tea, and energy drinks, as well as alcoholic beverages, particularly if you notice they exacerbate your symptoms.

Histamine, Rich Foods:

Histamine is a compound that is naturally produced by the body and can also be found in certain foods. In individuals with sinusitis, consuming foods high in histamine can trigger allergic reactions or worsen existing symptoms. Some examples of histamine, rich foods include aged cheeses, cured meats, fermented foods, and certain types of fish. Pay attention to how your body reacts to these foods and consider avoiding or reducing them if necessary.

Spicy Foods:

While spicy foods can provide temporary relief by clearing nasal passages, they can also irritate the sinuses and cause inflammation in some individuals. Pay attention to your body's response to spicy foods and avoid them if they exacerbate your sinusitis symptoms.

Gluten and Wheat Products:

Some individuals with sinusitis may have sensitivities or allergies to gluten or wheat, which can lead to inflammation and worsen sinus symptoms. If you suspect gluten or wheat intolerance, consider eliminating or reducing gluten and wheat products from your diet and observe how your symptoms respond.

Allergenic Foods:

Certain foods have the potential to trigger allergic reactions in susceptible individuals, leading to worsened sinusitis symptoms. Common allergenic foods include peanuts, tree nuts, shellfish, eggs, soy, and wheat. If you have known food allergies or suspect that certain foods are triggering your symptoms, it is advisable to avoid those foods or seek medical advice.

Artificial Additives and Preservatives:

Foods containing artificial additives, preservatives, and colorings may exacerbate inflammation and contribute to overall poor health. These additives can be found in processed foods, sodas, snack foods, and fast food. Reading food labels and choosing whole, natural foods can help you avoid these potentially problematic additives.

Hydration and Sinus Health

Hydration and Sinus Health: The Importance of Adequate Fluid Intake for Sinusitis Relief

When it comes to managing sinusitis, a condition characterized by inflammation or infection of the sinuses, proper hydration is often overlooked but plays a crucial role in maintaining sinus health and alleviating symptoms. Staying adequately hydrated helps thin mucus secretions, promote sinus drainage, and prevent dehydration, which can worsen sinusitis symptoms. Below we will explore the relationship between hydration and sinus health and discuss the importance of adequate fluid intake in managing sinusitis effectively.

Thin Mucus Secretions:

Sinusitis often leads to thickened mucus in the sinus cavities, causing congestion and discomfort. Drinking sufficient fluids helps thin the mucus, making it easier to expel and facilitating nasal drainage. When mucus is thin and flowing properly, it reduces the likelihood of blockages and helps alleviate congestion.

Promote Sinus Drainage:

Proper hydration is essential for promoting sinus drainage, which is crucial for clearing mucus and preventing the buildup of bacteria and irritants in the sinuses. Drinking an adequate amount of fluids helps maintain the necessary moisture in the sinus membranes, allowing them to function optimally and facilitate drainage.

Relieve Sinus Pressure and Congestion:

Dehydration can lead to thickened mucus, causing increased sinus pressure and congestion. By ensuring adequate hydration, you can help prevent the thickening of mucus and alleviate sinus pressure, providing relief from discomfort and congestion associated with sinusitis.

Optimal Immune Function:

Adequate hydration is vital for supporting a healthy immune system, which plays a crucial role in fighting off infections and reducing inflammation. When the body is well, hydrated, it can better defend against pathogens and maintain optimal immune function, reducing the likelihood of developing sinusitis or other respiratory infections.

Moisturize Sinus Passages:

Dry air can exacerbate sinusitis symptoms and cause discomfort. By staying hydrated, you can help moisturize the nasal passages and sinuses, providing relief from dryness and irritation. This is particularly important in dry environments or during seasons when indoor heating or air conditioning can contribute to dry sinus passages.

Prevention of Dehydration:

Dehydration can worsen sinusitis symptoms and contribute to overall discomfort. When the body is dehydrated, the mucus membranes can become dry and less effective at trapping and eliminating irritants, bacteria, and allergens. This can lead to increased susceptibility to infections and prolonged sinusitis symptoms. Adequate hydration helps prevent dehydration and promotes optimal sinus health.

Recommendations for Fluid Intake:

While fluid needs may vary depending on factors such as age, activity level, and overall health, a general guideline for fluid intake is to aim for around 8 cups (64 ounces) of fluids per day. This can include water, herbal teas, clear broths, and other hydrating beverages. Additionally, consuming fluids through hydrating foods like fruits and vegetables can contribute to overall hydration.

Tips for Staying Hydrated:

Carry a reusable water bottle with you throughout the day as a reminder to drink water regularly.

Set reminders on your phone or use apps that help track and remind you to drink water.

Flavor water with slices of citrus fruits, cucumbers, or berries to enhance its taste and make it more enticing to drink.

Drink water before, during, and after physical activity or exposure to dry environments.

Consume hydrating foods such as watermelon, cucumber, oranges, and celery, which have high water content.

Limit the intake of dehydrating beverages such as caffeinated and alcoholic drinks, as they can have diuretic effects.

Chapter Sixteen

Understanding Allergies and Sinusitis

Understanding Allergies and Sinusitis: Exploring the Connection and Managing Symptoms

Sinusitis and allergies are two distinct conditions, but they often go hand in hand. Allergies can be a contributing factor to the development of sinusitis or exacerbate its symptoms. Below we will explore the connection between allergies and sinusitis, understand the underlying mechanisms, and discuss effective strategies for managing symptoms and improving quality of life.

The Link Between Allergies and Sinusitis:

Sinusitis refers to inflammation or infection of the sinuses, which are hollow spaces in the skull that are connected to the nasal passages. Allergies, on the other hand, occur when the immune system overreacts to harmless substances such as pollen, dust mites, pet dander, or certain foods. Allergens trigger an immune response, leading to symptoms like sneezing, itching, nasal congestion, and inflammation.

Allergic Rhinitis and Sinusitis:

Allergic rhinitis, commonly known as hay fever, is a type of allergy that affects the nasal passages. When allergens such as pollen or dust come into contact with the nasal lining, they can cause inflammation and trigger symptoms similar to sinusitis, including congestion, nasal discharge, facial pain, and pressure. If left untreated, allergic rhinitis can contribute to the development of sinusitis.

Underlying Mechanisms:

Allergic reactions involve the release of histamine and other chemicals by immune cells, resulting in inflammation and increased mucus production. In individuals with allergic rhinitis, prolonged exposure to allergens can lead to chronic inflammation in the nasal passages, impairing the natural defense mechanisms of the sinuses and increasing the risk of sinusitis.

Allergies as a Trigger for Acute Sinusitis:

Acute sinusitis can be triggered or worsened by allergies. When the nasal passages are inflamed due to allergies, they become swollen and congested, impeding the drainage of mucus from the sinuses. This blockage creates a favorable environment for bacteria to grow, leading to the development of acute sinusitis.

Chronic Rhinosinusitis:

Chronic rhinosinusitis is a condition characterized by persistent inflammation of the nasal passages and sinuses lasting for more than 12 weeks. Allergies can be a significant contributing factor to the development of chronic rhinosinusitis. Prolonged exposure to allergens can cause ongoing inflammation, impair the normal functioning of the sinuses, and lead to persistent symptoms.

Managing Allergies and Sinusitis:

Effective management of allergies is crucial for preventing or reducing the occurrence of sinusitis. Here are some strategies to consider:

Identify and avoid allergens: If you know the specific allergens that trigger your symptoms, take steps to minimize your exposure to them. This may involve keeping windows closed during high pollen seasons, using allergen, proof covers for bedding, and avoiding contact with pets or other sources of allergens.

Use nasal saline rinses: Nasal saline rinses can help flush out allergens and reduce nasal inflammation. They are particularly useful for individuals with allergic rhinitis or those prone to sinusitis. Saline rinses can be done using a neti pot or squeeze bottle filled with a saline solution.

Consider allergy medications: Over, the, counter antihistamines, nasal corticosteroids, and decongestants can provide relief from allergy symptoms and reduce inflammation in the nasal passages. However, it's important to consult with a healthcare professional before starting any medication.

Immunotherapy: For individuals with severe allergies or those whose symptoms are not adequately controlled by medications, allergen immunotherapy may be recommended.

Common Allergens

Unveiling Common Allergens: Understanding Their Impact on Sinusitis

Sinusitis, a condition characterized by inflammation or infection of the sinuses, can be triggered or exacerbated by exposure to certain allergens. Identifying and understanding common allergens is crucial for managing sinusitis effectively and minimizing symptoms. Below we will explore some of the most common allergens and their potential impact on sinusitis, shedding light on ways to minimize exposure and alleviate symptoms.

Pollen:

Pollen is one of the most prevalent allergens, and it can trigger symptoms of sinusitis in susceptible individuals. It is released by trees, grasses, and weeds during certain seasons, leading to allergic rhinitis or hay fever. Common symptoms include sneezing, itching, nasal congestion, and sinus pressure. Monitoring pollen levels and taking appropriate precautions, such as keeping windows closed during high pollen seasons or using air purifiers, can help minimize exposure.

Dust Mites:

Dust mites are microscopic organisms commonly found in bedding, carpets, and upholstered furniture. Their waste products can trigger allergic reactions and worsen sinusitis symptoms. Reducing exposure to dust mites involves regular washing of bedding in hot water, using allergen, proof covers on mattresses and pillows, and keeping the home clean and well, ventilated.

Pet Dander:

Animal dander, including the skin cells, saliva, and urine of pets, can act as a potent allergen for many people. Cats and dogs are the most common culprits, but other animals such as birds, rabbits, and rodents can also trigger allergies. Avoiding direct contact with pets, keeping them out of bedrooms, and regularly cleaning surfaces and furniture can help reduce exposure to pet dander.

Mold Spores:

Mold spores are airborne particles released by molds that grow in damp environments, such as bathrooms, basements, and kitchens. Inhalation of mold spores can cause allergic reactions and contribute to sinusitis symptoms. Preventing mold growth by controlling moisture levels, ensuring proper ventilation, and promptly addressing any water leaks or dampness is essential in minimizing exposure.

Cockroaches:

Cockroach droppings, saliva, and body parts contain allergenic proteins that can trigger allergies and worsen sinusitis symptoms. Cockroach infestations are more common in urban areas and can be challenging to eradicate. Minimizing exposure to cockroaches involves keeping the home clean, sealing cracks and crevices, and promptly addressing any signs of infestation.

Tree Nuts:

While tree nut allergies primarily affect the digestive and immune systems, they can also contribute to sinusitis symptoms in susceptible individuals. Ingesting or inhaling particles of tree nuts can trigger an allergic reaction, causing nasal congestion, sneezing, and facial pressure. Those with tree nut allergies should strictly avoid consuming tree nuts and be cautious of cross, contamination.

Shellfish:

Shellfish allergies, particularly to crustaceans such as shrimp, crab, and lobster, can cause allergic reactions that affect the respiratory system. Inhaling steam or cooking fumes from shellfish can trigger symptoms of sinusitis, including nasal congestion and inflammation. Avoiding shellfish and being vigilant about cross, contamination in food preparation can help minimize exposure.

Latex:

Latex allergies can develop after repeated exposure to latex, containing products such as gloves, balloons, or medical devices. Inhalation of latex particles can lead to sinusitis symptoms in sensitized individuals. Substituting latex products with latex, free alternatives and informing healthcare professionals about latex allergies before medical procedures is crucial in preventing reactions.

Allergy Testing

Allergy Testing: Unlocking the Key to Managing Sinusitis

Sinusitis, characterized by inflammation or infection of the sinuses, can often be triggered or worsened by allergies. Allergy testing plays a vital role in identifying specific allergens that contribute to sinusitis symptoms. By pinpointing the triggers, individuals can take proactive measures to manage their condition effectively. Below we will explore the significance of allergy testing in relation to sinusitis and shed light on various testing methods available.

Understanding Allergy Testing:

Allergy testing is a diagnostic tool used to determine the specific substances or allergens that trigger an individual's allergic reactions. These tests can help identify allergens that may be contributing to sinusitis symptoms, allowing for targeted management strategies.

Signs that May Indicate the Need for Allergy Testing:

If an individual experiences recurring or persistent sinusitis symptoms, such as nasal congestion, sneezing, facial pressure, or headaches, despite appropriate medical treatment, allergy testing may be recommended. Other indicators include a family history of allergies or a known sensitivity to certain substances.

Types of Allergy Testing:

There are two main types of allergy testing: skin tests and blood tests.

a) Skin Tests:

Skin tests involve the introduction of small amounts of allergens into the skin to observe the body's reaction. The two most common types of skin tests are:

Skin prick test: In this test, a small amount of allergen extract is pricked onto the skin's surface, usually on the forearm or back. If a person is allergic to the specific allergen, a localized reaction, such as redness, swelling, or itching, will occur.

Intradermal test: Intradermal testing involves injecting a small amount of allergen extract into the skin's deeper layers. This test is typically used when the results of the skin prick test are inconclusive or further investigation is needed.

b) Blood Tests:

Blood tests measure the presence of specific antibodies in the blood that are associated with allergic reactions. The two primary types of blood tests are:

Enzyme, linked immunosorbent assay (ELISA): This test measures the level of allergen, specific antibodies, known as immunoglobulin E (IgE), in the blood. It can provide valuable information about an individual's sensitization to specific allergens.

Radioallergosorbent test (RAST): RAST is another blood test that detects specific IgE antibodies in response to particular allergens. It is often used when skin testing is not feasible or contraindicated.

Benefits of Allergy Testing for Sinusitis:

Allergy testing offers several advantages in managing sinusitis:

Identifying specific allergens: Testing helps pinpoint the exact substances that trigger allergic reactions, providing valuable information for targeted avoidance strategies.

Customized treatment plans: Knowing the specific allergens allows healthcare providers to develop personalized treatment plans, including allergen avoidance measures, medications, and immunotherapy.

Minimizing unnecessary medication use: By identifying the root cause of sinusitis symptoms, allergy testing can reduce reliance on medications that only alleviate symptoms without addressing the underlying allergen triggers.

Preventing future exacerbations: Allergy testing helps individuals proactively manage their condition by implementing preventive measures to avoid allergen exposure, minimizing the risk of recurrent sinusitis episodes.

Preparing for Allergy Testing:

Communicate with your healthcare provider: Provide a comprehensive medical history, including any known allergies or reactions to substances.

Medication adjustments: Some medications, such as antihistamines, can interfere with allergy test results. Your healthcare provider may advise discontinuing certain medications for a specified period before testing.

Allergy Treatments

Allergy Treatments: Empowering Individuals in the Management of Sinusitis

Sinusitis, characterized by inflammation or infection of the sinuses, can often be triggered or worsened by allergies. Effective allergy treatments play a crucial role in managing sinusitis symptoms and improving quality of life. Below we will explore various treatment options available for allergies and their relevance to sinusitis, empowering individuals to make informed decisions about their healthcare.

Allergy Medications:

Allergy medications are often the first line of defense in managing sinusitis symptoms caused by allergens. They aim to alleviate symptoms by reducing inflammation, suppressing the immune response, and blocking the effects of histamine. Common allergy medications include:

Antihistamines: These medications counteract the effects of histamine, a chemical released during an allergic reaction. They can help relieve sneezing, itching, runny nose, and watery eyes.

Nasal corticosteroids: These nasal sprays reduce inflammation in the nasal passages, relieving congestion and nasal symptoms associated with allergies and sinusitis.

Decongestants: Decongestants work by shrinking the blood vessels in the nasal passages, reducing swelling and congestion. They provide temporary relief from nasal congestion but should be used cautiously due to potential side effects.

Leukotriene modifiers: These medications block the action of leukotrienes, chemicals released during an allergic reaction that contribute to inflammation and mucus production.

Mast cell stabilizers: Mast cell stabilizers prevent the release of histamine and other inflammatory chemicals from immune cells, helping to control allergic reactions.

Immunotherapy:

Immunotherapy, also known as allergy shots or allergy desensitization, is a long, term treatment option for individuals with severe allergies. It involves regular injections of allergen extracts to help the body gradually build tolerance to specific allergens. Immunotherapy aims to modify the immune response, reduce sensitivity to allergens, and alleviate allergy symptoms, including those related to sinusitis.

Subcutaneous immunotherapy (SCIT): SCIT involves injecting allergen extracts into the fatty tissue under the skin. The treatment is administered in increasing doses over a period of several months, followed by a maintenance phase. SCIT can be effective in reducing allergy symptoms and preventing the development of sinusitis.

Sublingual immunotherapy (SLIT): SLIT involves placing allergen extracts under the tongue, where they are absorbed into the bloodstream. SLIT is typically administered in the form of tablets or drops. It can be a convenient and effective alternative to SCIT, especially for individuals who cannot tolerate injections.

Benefits of immunotherapy: Immunotherapy aims to provide long, term relief by targeting the underlying cause of allergies rather than just managing symptoms. It can significantly reduce the need for medication, improve quality of life, and potentially prevent the progression of sinusitis.

Nasal Irrigation:

Nasal irrigation, also known as nasal rinsing or nasal saline irrigation, is a technique that involves flushing the nasal passages with a saline solution. It can help relieve sinusitis symptoms by rinsing away allergens, mucus, and irritants from the nasal passages, promoting nasal health and reducing inflammation.

Neti pots: Neti pots are small vessels used to pour saline solution into one nostril, allowing it to flow out through the other nostril, flushing the sinuses. They can be an effective way to alleviate congestion and improve sinus drainage.

Nasal irrigation devices: Nasal irrigation devices, such as squeeze bottles or nasal irrigation kits, provide a controlled flow of saline solution to flush the nasal passages. They offer convenience and ease of use compared to traditional neti pots.

Chapter Seventeen

The Future of Sinusitis Treatment

The Future of Sinusitis Treatment: Pioneering Advancements on the Horizon

Sinusitis, a condition characterized by inflammation or infection of the sinuses, affects millions of people worldwide. While current treatment options provide relief for many individuals, ongoing research and advancements in medical technology offer promising prospects for the future of sinusitis treatment. Below we will explore some of the exciting developments and innovations that may revolutionize the management of sinusitis in the years to come.

Precision Medicine:

Precision medicine, also known as personalized medicine, is an emerging approach that tailors medical treatment to an individual's specific characteristics, including their genetic makeup, environmental factors, and lifestyle. This approach holds significant potential for sinusitis treatment by enabling healthcare professionals to customize therapies based on an individual's unique needs and underlying causes of the condition.

Genetic testing: Genetic testing may help identify genetic factors that contribute to sinusitis susceptibility or treatment response. Understanding an individual's genetic profile could aid in predicting their risk of developing sinusitis and guiding targeted interventions.

Biomarkers: Research is underway to identify specific biomarkers associated with sinusitis. Biomarkers are measurable indicators, such as proteins or genetic markers, that can provide insights into disease progression, response to treatment, and individualized management strategies.

Biologic Therapies:

Biologic therapies are medications derived from living organisms or produced using genetic engineering techniques. These innovative treatments target specific molecules or cells involved in the inflammatory process, aiming to restore immune balance and alleviate sinusitis symptoms. Biologic therapies currently used in other conditions, such as asthma or rheumatoid arthritis, are being investigated for their potential in managing chronic sinusitis.

Monoclonal antibodies: Monoclonal antibodies are laboratory, produced antibodies designed to bind to specific targets in the immune system. They can block inflammatory pathways and reduce the severity of sinusitis symptoms.

Cytokine inhibitors: Cytokines are proteins involved in immune responses and inflammation. Inhibiting specific cytokines, such as interleukins or tumor necrosis factor, may help modulate the immune response and alleviate sinusitis symptoms.

Growth factors: Growth factors promote tissue repair and regeneration. Utilizing growth factors to stimulate healing in the sinus lining may help restore normal sinus function and reduce the frequency and severity of sinusitis episodes.

Targeted Drug Delivery Systems:

Targeted drug delivery systems aim to deliver medications directly to the affected area, maximizing therapeutic effectiveness while minimizing systemic side effects. Researchers are exploring various approaches to enhance drug delivery to the sinuses, including:

Intranasal nanoparticles: Nanoparticles are tiny particles that can carry medications and deliver them directly to the sinus tissues. They can improve drug absorption and prolong the therapeutic effect, leading to more efficient symptom relief.

Drug, eluting implants: Implantable devices, such as stents or sinus implants, can be placed during sinus surgery to deliver medication directly to the sinuses over an extended period. These devices can provide sustained drug release, reducing the need for frequent medication administration.

Minimally Invasive Procedures:

Minimally invasive procedures aim to treat sinusitis with minimal disruption to the surrounding tissues, leading to faster recovery times, reduced pain, and improved outcomes. Several innovative techniques are being developed to address various aspects of sinusitis management:

Balloon sinuplasty: Balloon sinuplasty is a minimally invasive procedure that uses a small balloon catheter to gently widen the sinus openings, promoting better drainage and airflow. It offers a less invasive alternative to traditional sinus surgery and can be performed on an outpatient basis.

Advances in Sinus Surgery

Advances in Sinus Surgery: Pioneering Techniques for Effective Sinusitis Treatment

Sinusitis, a condition characterized by inflammation or infection of the sinuses, can cause significant discomfort and impact the quality of life for millions of individuals worldwide. While medical therapies provide relief for many, advances in surgical techniques have revolutionized the management of sinusitis. Below we will explore the innovative surgical approaches that have emerged, offering more effective and long, lasting solutions for sinusitis treatment.

Endoscopic Sinus Surgery:

Endoscopic sinus surgery is a minimally invasive procedure that utilizes an endoscope, a thin, flexible tube with a camera on the end, to visualize and access the sinuses. It allows surgeons to precisely remove obstructions, inflamed tissue, and polyps, promoting better sinus drainage and airflow. Endoscopic sinus surgery offers several benefits over traditional open surgery, including:

Reduced trauma and scarring: The procedure is performed through the nostrils, eliminating the need for external incisions. This results in less tissue damage, reduced scarring, and a faster recovery time.

Improved visualization: The endoscope provides high, definition images of the sinuses, allowing surgeons to navigate and treat the affected areas with enhanced precision.

Preservation of normal anatomy: The targeted removal of diseased tissue helps preserve the natural structure of the sinuses, minimizing the risk of complications and promoting better long, term outcomes.

Image, Guided Navigation Systems:

Image, guided navigation systems are advanced technologies that integrate real, time imaging, such as computed tomography (CT) scans, with surgical instruments. These systems provide surgeons with detailed 3D maps of the sinus anatomy during surgery, allowing for more accurate and precise interventions. Key benefits of image, guided navigation systems include:

Enhanced precision: Surgeons can precisely identify and navigate the complex sinus anatomy, ensuring targeted treatment and reducing the risk of complications.

Improved safety: The real, time imaging feedback helps surgeons avoid critical structures, such as the eyes or brain, minimizing the risk of damage during the procedure.

Extended reach: Image, guided navigation systems enable access to hard, to, reach areas of the sinuses, ensuring thorough treatment and reducing the likelihood of disease recurrence.

Balloon Sinuplasty:

Balloon sinuplasty is a minimally invasive procedure that utilizes a small balloon catheter to gently dilate the sinus openings, restoring proper drainage and airflow. The procedure is typically performed under local anesthesia and offers several advantages:

Reduced tissue trauma: Unlike traditional surgery, balloon sinuplasty does not involve tissue removal or cutting. The gentle dilation of the sinus openings minimizes tissue trauma and promotes faster healing.

Shorter recovery time: Due to its minimally invasive nature, patients typically experience less pain, swelling, and bleeding after balloon sinuplasty. This results in a quicker recovery and a faster return to normal activities.

Outpatient procedure: Balloon sinuplasty can often be performed on an outpatient basis, allowing patients to undergo the procedure and return home the same day.

Robotic, Assisted Sinus Surgery:

Robotic, assisted sinus surgery combines the precision of robotics with the expertise of the surgeon. The surgeon controls a robotic arm equipped with miniature instruments, allowing for enhanced dexterity and accuracy during the procedure. Robotic, assisted sinus surgery offers several benefits:

Enhanced visualization: The high, definition 3D imaging provided by the robotic system enables surgeons to visualize the sinus anatomy in detail, enhancing precision and reducing the risk of complications.

Greater flexibility: The robotic system allows for increased maneuverability and access to challenging areas of the sinuses, ensuring comprehensive treatment.

New Medications

New Medications: Transforming the Treatment of Sinusitis

Sinusitis, a condition characterized by inflammation or infection of the sinuses, can cause significant discomfort and impact the quality of life for millions of individuals worldwide. While traditional treatments such as antibiotics, nasal sprays, and decongestants have been the mainstay of sinusitis management, ongoing research and development have led to the emergence of new medications that offer innovative approaches and improved outcomes. Below we will explore some of the exciting advancements in medication therapy that are transforming the treatment of sinusitis.

Topical Steroids:

Topical steroids, also known as corticosteroids, have long been used in the management of sinusitis. However, recent developments have led to the introduction of more advanced formulations that offer enhanced efficacy and convenience.

Nasal steroid sprays: Nasal steroid sprays deliver corticosteroids directly to the nasal passages, reducing inflammation and swelling. Newer formulations provide improved nasal delivery, longer duration of action, and better patient compliance.

Nasal irrigations: Nasal irrigations with steroid solutions allow for a more targeted and controlled delivery of medication to the sinuses. This approach helps reduce inflammation and promote sinus drainage, providing relief from symptoms.

Antifungal Medications:

Fungal sinusitis, a specific type of sinusitis caused by fungal infections, poses unique challenges in treatment. New antifungal medications have been developed to target the specific fungal pathogens involved, improving outcomes for patients with fungal sinusitis.

Oral antifungal agents: Oral antifungal medications, such as voriconazole or itraconazole, have demonstrated efficacy in treating fungal sinusitis. These medications target the underlying fungal infection and help alleviate symptoms.

Antifungal nasal sprays: Antifungal nasal sprays deliver medication directly to the nasal passages, targeting the fungal infection in the sinuses. These sprays may be used as an adjunct to oral antifungal therapy or as a standalone treatment for milder cases of fungal sinusitis.

Immunomodulators:

Immunomodulators are medications that help regulate and balance the immune response. They have shown promise in managing chronic sinusitis by addressing underlying immune dysfunction and reducing inflammation.

Immunotherapy: Immunotherapy, also known as allergy shots, is a treatment approach that aims to desensitize the immune system to specific allergens. By gradually exposing the body to small amounts of the allergen, immunotherapy helps retrain the immune system and reduce allergic reactions that contribute to sinusitis symptoms.

Biological response modifiers: Biological response modifiers are a class of medications that target specific molecules or pathways involved in the immune response. They help modulate the immune system and reduce inflammation associated with chronic sinusitis.

Mucolytic Agents:

Mucolytic agents are medications that help thin and loosen mucus, making it easier to expel from the sinuses. These agents can improve sinus drainage and alleviate congestion.

Expectorants: Expectorants are oral medications that promote mucus clearance by increasing the production of thin, watery mucus. This helps prevent mucus from becoming thick and sticky, facilitating its removal from the sinuses.

Mucolytic enzymes: Mucolytic enzymes, such as bromelain or N, acetylcysteine, help break down the proteins present in thick mucus, making it less viscous and easier to clear.

Probiotics:

Probiotics, also known as "good bacteria," have gained attention for their potential role in promoting immune health and reducing inflammation. Studies have suggested that probiotics may have a positive impact on sinusitis by balancing the microbiome and supporting immune function.

Emerging Therapies

Emerging Therapies: Shaping the Future of Sinusitis Treatment

Sinusitis, a condition characterized by inflammation or infection of the sinuses, can significantly impact the quality of life for individuals. While traditional treatments have provided relief for many, ongoing research and development have led to the emergence of innovative therapies that offer promising new approaches for sinusitis management. Below we will explore some of the exciting emerging therapies that are shaping the future of sinusitis treatment.

Biologics:

Biologics are a class of medications derived from living organisms that target specific molecules or pathways involved in the inflammatory process. They offer a targeted and personalized approach to sinusitis treatment by addressing the underlying immune dysfunction and reducing inflammation.

Monoclonal antibodies: Monoclonal antibodies are engineered proteins that target specific inflammatory molecules. They can help modulate the immune response and reduce inflammation in chronic sinusitis. Studies have shown promising results in terms of symptom improvement and reduction in disease recurrence.

Cytokine inhibitors: Cytokines are small proteins involved in the immune response and inflammation. Inhibitors of specific cytokines, such as interleukin, 4 (IL, 4) or interleukin, 13 (IL, 13), have shown efficacy in reducing inflammation and improving symptoms in patients with chronic sinusitis.

Antimicrobial Peptides:

Antimicrobial peptides (AMPs) are naturally occurring molecules that have antimicrobial properties. They can target and kill bacteria, viruses, and fungi without causing resistance. AMPs offer a potential alternative to traditional antibiotics in the treatment of sinusitis, especially in cases of recurrent or antibiotic, resistant infections.

Synthetic AMPs: Researchers are developing synthetic versions of naturally occurring AMPs, which can be delivered directly to the sinuses to combat infection. These synthetic AMPs have shown efficacy against a broad range of pathogens, including drug, resistant strains.

Photodynamic Therapy:

Photodynamic therapy (PDT) is a treatment approach that combines the use of a photosensitizing agent and light activation to destroy bacteria and reduce inflammation. PDT has shown promise in the management of chronic sinusitis by targeting the underlying infection and promoting healing.

Photosensitizing agents: Photosensitizing agents are applied to the sinus lining and selectively absorbed by bacteria. When activated by light of a specific wavelength, these agents generate reactive oxygen species that destroy bacteria and reduce inflammation.

Light activation: Light of the appropriate wavelength is delivered to the sinuses to activate the photosensitizing agent. The light can be administered using fiber, optic devices, ensuring precise targeting of the affected areas.

Stem Cell Therapy:

Stem cell therapy holds potential for regenerative medicine in various fields, including sinusitis treatment. Researchers are exploring the use of stem cells to repair damaged sinus tissues and promote healing.

Mesenchymal stem cells: Mesenchymal stem cells (MSCs) are a type of adult stem cell that can differentiate into various cell types and possess anti, inflammatory properties. MSCs can be harvested from a patient's own bone marrow or adipose tissue and then delivered to the sinuses to promote tissue regeneration and reduce inflammation.

Tissue engineering: Tissue engineering approaches involve the use of scaffolds seeded with stem cells to regenerate damaged sinus tissues. These scaffolds provide structural support and guidance for tissue growth, facilitating the repair process.

Gene Therapy:

Gene therapy involves the transfer of genetic material into cells to modify their function and restore normal cellular processes. In the context of sinusitis, gene therapy aims to correct underlying genetic defects or modulate immune responses to reduce inflammation.

Chapter Eighteen

Living with Sinusitis

Living with Sinusitis: Navigating the Challenges and Seeking Relief

Sinusitis, a condition characterized by inflammation or infection of the sinuses, can significantly impact the quality of life for those affected. The symptoms of sinusitis, such as nasal congestion, facial pain, and pressure, can be debilitating and affect various aspects of daily life. Below we will explore the challenges faced by individuals living with sinusitis and discuss strategies for managing the condition and seeking relief.

Understanding the Impact:

Living with sinusitis can present numerous challenges that extend beyond the physical symptoms. The persistent discomfort and pain can lead to fatigue, decreased productivity, and diminished overall well, being. The impact on mental health should not be overlooked, as individuals with chronic sinusitis may experience frustration, anxiety, and even depression due to the prolonged nature of the condition.

Treatment Approaches:

The management of sinusitis involves a multifaceted approach aimed at alleviating symptoms and preventing recurrent episodes. It is important for individuals with sinusitis to work closely with healthcare professionals to develop an individualized treatment plan. This may include:

Medications: Depending on the severity and underlying causes of sinusitis, various medications may be prescribed, such as antibiotics to treat bacterial infections, nasal sprays to reduce inflammation, and pain relievers to alleviate discomfort.

Allergy management: Allergies can often exacerbate sinusitis symptoms. Identifying and avoiding allergens through allergen testing and implementing allergy management strategies can help reduce the frequency and severity of sinusitis episodes.

Nasal irrigation: Regular nasal irrigation using saline solutions can help clear mucus and reduce inflammation, providing relief from congestion and facilitating sinus drainage.

Steam inhalation: Steam inhalation can help moisturize the nasal passages, alleviate congestion, and promote sinus drainage. Adding essential oils, such as eucalyptus or peppermint, to the steam can further enhance the therapeutic benefits.

Lifestyle Modifications:

In addition to medical interventions, certain lifestyle modifications can help individuals better manage their sinusitis symptoms and improve their overall well, being.

Environmental control: Creating a clean and allergen, free environment can significantly reduce sinusitis symptoms. Regularly cleaning and dusting the living space, using air purifiers, and minimizing exposure to irritants like tobacco smoke and strong odors can make a noticeable difference.

Humidification: Maintaining appropriate humidity levels in the living environment is important for sinus health. Using humidifiers or vaporizers can help keep the nasal passages moist and prevent excessive dryness, which can worsen sinusitis symptoms.

Regular exercise: Engaging in regular physical exercise not only helps boost overall health but can also enhance the immune system and improve sinus drainage. Moderate exercise, such as walking or swimming, can be beneficial in managing sinusitis.

Stress management: Stress can exacerbate sinusitis symptoms and weaken the immune system. Employing stress management techniques such as yoga, meditation, deep breathing exercises, or engaging in hobbies can help reduce stress levels and promote overall well, being.

Seeking Support:

Living with sinusitis can be challenging, both physically and emotionally. Seeking support from healthcare professionals, support groups, and loved ones can provide valuable guidance, understanding, and encouragement.

Healthcare professionals: Regular communication with healthcare professionals can ensure appropriate management of sinusitis and adjustment of treatment plans as needed. They can provide education, monitor progress, and offer additional therapeutic options when required.

Support groups: Joining support groups or online communities dedicated to sinusitis can provide a sense of belonging and a platform to share experiences and coping strategies. Interacting with others who face similar challenges can be empowering and help individuals feel less alone in their journey.

Managing Symptoms

Managing Symptoms of Sinusitis: Strategies for Relief and Comfort

Sinusitis, a condition characterized by inflammation or infection of the sinuses, can cause a range of bothersome symptoms that affect daily life.

From nasal congestion and facial pressure to headaches and fatigue, the symptoms of sinusitis can be frustrating and challenging to manage. Below we will explore various strategies for effectively managing the symptoms of sinusitis, providing relief and improving overall comfort.

Nasal Irrigation:

Nasal irrigation, also known as nasal rinsing or sinus irrigation, is a simple yet effective technique that helps alleviate sinusitis symptoms. It involves flushing out the nasal passages with a saline solution to remove excess mucus, reduce inflammation, and promote better sinus drainage.

Neti pot: Using a neti pot, a small vessel shaped like a teapot, allows for controlled pouring of the saline solution into one nostril while tilting the head to let the solution flow out through the other nostril. This process helps clear the sinuses and provides relief from congestion.

Nasal irrigation kits: Various nasal irrigation kits, such as squeeze bottles or bulb syringes, are available for those who prefer a different approach. These kits provide a convenient way to deliver the saline solution into the nasal passages, flushing out irritants and promoting better breathing.

Steam Inhalation:

Steam inhalation is a time, tested home remedy that can provide immediate relief from sinusitis symptoms. The warm, moist air helps soothe irritated nasal passages, reduce congestion, and promote sinus drainage.

Hot shower or bath: Taking a hot shower or bath allows the steam to fill the bathroom, creating a humid environment that helps moisturize the nasal passages. Spending a few minutes in the steam can provide temporary relief and make breathing easier.

Steam bowl: Boiling water in a bowl and leaning over it while placing a towel over the head creates a makeshift steam tent. Inhaling the steam through the nose helps moisten the nasal passages and loosen mucus, providing relief from congestion.

Warm Compress:

A warm compress applied to the face can help alleviate facial pain, pressure, and discomfort associated with sinusitis. The heat improves blood circulation, reduces inflammation, and provides soothing relief.

Warm towel: Soaking a clean towel in warm water and wringing out the excess moisture creates a warm compress. Gently placing the warm towel over the affected sinus areas for a few minutes can help alleviate pain and promote relaxation.

Warm pack or heating pad: Using a commercially available warm pack or heating pad designed for the face provides a consistent and controlled level of warmth. Applying the warm pack to the affected areas can provide targeted relief and enhance comfort.

Saline Nasal Sprays:

Saline nasal sprays are over, the, counter products that contain a saltwater solution. They can help moisturize the nasal passages, relieve dryness, and flush out irritants, providing temporary relief from congestion and promoting sinus health.

Application technique: Using a saline nasal spray involves inserting the nozzle into one nostril while tilting the head slightly forward. A gentle squeeze of the bottle delivers a fine mist of the saline solution into the nasal passage. The process is repeated for the other nostril.

Frequency of use: Saline nasal sprays are safe for regular use and can be applied multiple times a day, as needed. They can provide instant relief and help maintain nasal moisture, reducing the severity of symptoms.

Over, the, Counter Medications:

Certain over, the, counter medications can be helpful in managing sinusitis symptoms. However, it is important to consult with a healthcare professional before using any medication to ensure proper dosage and suitability for individual needs.

Staying Active

Embracing an Active Lifestyle: How Exercise Can Benefit Individuals with Sinusitis

Sinusitis, a condition characterized by inflammation or infection of the sinuses, can make physical activity challenging due to symptoms such as nasal congestion, facial pressure, and fatigue. However, staying active can have numerous benefits for individuals with sinusitis, including improved sinus health, enhanced overall well, being, and reduced symptom severity. Below we will explore the importance of staying active and provide insights into how exercise can positively impact individuals with sinusitis.

Enhancing Sinus Drainage:

Regular exercise plays a crucial role in promoting healthy sinus drainage. Physical activity helps increase blood circulation and lymphatic flow, which can aid in clearing mucus and reducing inflammation in the sinus cavities.

Cardiovascular exercise: Engaging in activities such as brisk walking, jogging, cycling, or swimming can help improve blood circulation throughout the body, including the nasal passages and sinuses. This increased circulation promotes efficient drainage and reduces congestion.

Yoga and stretching: Specific yoga poses and stretching exercises can target the neck, shoulders, and upper back, helping to relieve tension and pressure in the sinus areas. These gentle movements encourage sinus drainage and enhance overall comfort.

Boosting the Immune System:

Regular exercise has been shown to boost the immune system, which plays a crucial role in fighting off infections and reducing the severity of sinusitis symptoms.

Moderate, intensity exercise: Engaging in moderate, intensity exercise for at least 30 minutes most days of the week can strengthen the immune system. This can help reduce the frequency of sinusitis episodes and enhance the body's ability to recover from infections.

Outdoor activities: Exercising outdoors exposes individuals to fresh air and sunlight, which can have immune, boosting benefits. Spending time in nature, whether through activities like hiking, biking, or gardening, can provide a refreshing change of environment and promote overall well, being.

Managing Stress and Mental Health:

Sinusitis can take a toll on mental health, leading to increased stress levels and emotional strain. Regular exercise can help manage stress, improve mood, and enhance mental well, being.

Endorphin release: Exercise triggers the release of endorphins, often referred to as "feel, good" hormones. These endorphins can promote a sense of well, being, reduce stress, and improve overall mood.

Mind, body activities: Engaging in mind, body activities, such as yoga, tai chi, or Pilates, can have a calming effect on the mind and body. These activities combine physical movements with focused breathing and mindfulness, promoting relaxation and stress reduction.

Considerations for Exercising with Sinusitis:

While exercise offers numerous benefits for individuals with sinusitis, certain considerations should be kept in mind to ensure a safe and enjoyable experience.

Timing: It is important to listen to your body and choose the best time to exercise. Some individuals find that their sinus symptoms are more manageable in the morning, while others may prefer to exercise later in the day when symptoms have subsided. Find a time that works best for you.

Hydration: Staying hydrated before, during, and after exercise is crucial, as it helps thin mucus and prevents dehydration, which can worsen sinusitis symptoms. Be sure to drink plenty of water and consider carrying a water bottle during workouts.

Nasal protection: Individuals with sinusitis may find it helpful to use a saline nasal spray or perform nasal irrigation before exercise. This can help moisturize the nasal passages, reduce congestion, and facilitate better breathing during physical activity.

Gradual progression: If you are new to exercise or have been inactive due to sinusitis, it is important to start slowly and gradually increase the intensity and duration of your workouts.

Mental Health Considerations

Mental Health Considerations in Managing Sinusitis: Promoting Emotional Well, being Amidst Physical Discomfort

Sinusitis, a condition characterized by inflammation or infection of the sinuses, can take a toll not only on physical health but also on mental well, being. The persistent symptoms, such as facial pain, congestion, and fatigue, can lead to emotional distress, stress, and frustration. Below we will explore the mental health considerations associated with sinusitis and discuss strategies to promote emotional well, being while managing the physical discomfort.

Understanding the Emotional Impact of Sinusitis:

Living with chronic sinusitis can significantly impact an individual's mental health. The prolonged duration of symptoms, the uncertainty of flare, ups, and the impact on daily activities can contribute to various emotional challenges.

Frustration and irritability: Dealing with recurring symptoms can lead to frustration and irritability, as individuals may feel limited in their ability to participate in activities they enjoy or maintain their normal routines.

Anxiety and stress: The uncertainty and discomfort caused by sinusitis can trigger anxiety and stress. Worrying about the next flare, up, the impact on work or social engagements, and the overall management of the condition can take a toll on mental well, being.

Depression and mood changes: Living with chronic sinusitis can lead to feelings of sadness, hopelessness, or low mood. The constant presence of symptoms and the impact on daily life can contribute to a sense of despair or loss of enjoyment.

Seeking Emotional Support:

Managing sinusitis not only involves physical care but also requires attention to emotional well, being. Seeking support from healthcare professionals, friends, and family can make a significant difference in managing the mental health aspect of the condition.

Healthcare professionals: Open and honest communication with healthcare professionals is essential. They can provide guidance, offer treatment options, and address any concerns or questions related to sinusitis. They may also recommend additional support, such as counseling or therapy, to help manage the emotional impact.

Friends and family: Sharing experiences with trusted friends and family members can provide a source of empathy and understanding. They can offer emotional support, lend a listening ear, and provide encouragement during difficult times.

Coping Strategies for Emotional Well, being:

Implementing effective coping strategies can help individuals manage the emotional challenges associated with sinusitis and promote overall mental well, being.

Stress management techniques: Engaging in stress, reducing activities such as meditation, deep breathing exercises, and progressive muscle relaxation can help alleviate anxiety and promote a sense of calm. These techniques can be practiced regularly to manage stress levels.

Mindfulness practices: Incorporating mindfulness practices into daily life can help individuals stay present and manage negative emotions. Mindfulness exercises, such as mindful breathing or body scans, can bring awareness to the present moment and reduce excessive worrying or rumination.

Engaging in enjoyable activities: Despite the limitations caused by sinusitis, finding activities that bring joy and fulfillment is crucial for emotional well, being. Engaging in hobbies, creative outlets, or social interactions with loved ones can provide a sense of happiness and distract from the discomfort of sinusitis.

Balancing Rest and Activity:

Finding the right balance between rest and activity is essential in managing both the physical and mental aspects of sinusitis.

Prioritizing rest: Rest is crucial for the body's healing and recovery process. Ensuring an adequate amount of sleep and allowing oneself to rest when needed can contribute to overall well, being and reduce fatigue.

Gentle physical activity: While rest is important, engaging in gentle physical activity can have positive effects on mental health. Taking short walks, practicing gentle yoga, or engaging in light exercises can boost mood, improve energy levels, and promote a sense of well, being.

Chapter Nineteen

Resources and Support

Resources and Support: Navigating the Journey with Sinusitis

Living with sinusitis can be a challenging and sometimes isolating experience. The physical symptoms and emotional impact of the condition can take a toll on an individual's well, being. However, it's important to remember that you are not alone in this journey. Numerous resources and support systems are available to help you navigate the challenges of sinusitis and provide you with the information, guidance, and assistance you need. Below we will explore various resources and support options that can help you better manage sinusitis and enhance your overall quality of life.

Healthcare Professionals:

When dealing with sinusitis, your healthcare professionals are your primary source of support and guidance. They possess the knowledge and expertise to diagnose and treat your condition effectively. Here are some healthcare professionals who can play a role in your sinusitis management:

Primary care physician: Your primary care physician is often the first point of contact when experiencing sinusitis symptoms. They can provide initial evaluation, offer treatment options, and refer you to specialists if necessary.

Ear, Nose, and Throat (ENT) specialist: ENT specialists are experts in diagnosing and treating sinusitis. They can provide a more comprehensive evaluation of your sinuses, recommend appropriate treatments, and perform surgical interventions if needed.

Allergist: If your sinusitis is allergy, related, an allergist can help identify specific allergens that may be triggering your symptoms. They can conduct allergy testing, provide immunotherapy options, and assist in managing your allergies to reduce sinusitis flare, ups.

Online Resources:

The internet provides a wealth of information and resources for individuals with sinusitis. However, it's important to rely on reputable sources to ensure accurate and trustworthy information. Here are some online resources that can be helpful:

National Institutes of Health (NIH): The NIH website offers reliable information on sinusitis, including causes, symptoms, treatment options, and self, care strategies. It also provides access to relevant research articles and clinical trials.

Medical professional organizations: Websites of professional organizations, such as the American Academy of Otolaryngology, Head and Neck Surgery (AAO, HNS), provide comprehensive information on sinusitis, treatment guidelines, and educational materials for patients.

Health forums and support groups: Online communities dedicated to sinusitis can provide a platform for individuals to connect, share experiences, and seek advice. These forums can offer emotional support, practical tips, and personal insights from others living with sinusitis.

Supportive Networks:

Building a network of support can make a significant difference in your sinusitis journey. Here are some avenues for connecting with others facing similar challenges:

Local support groups: Seek out local support groups or meetups focused on sinusitis or related conditions. These gatherings allow you to connect with individuals who understand your experiences, share coping strategies, and provide a supportive environment.

Online support communities: Joining online support communities, such as social media groups or forums dedicated to sinusitis, can offer a virtual space for sharing experiences, asking questions, and receiving support from a global community of individuals.

Lifestyle and Self, Care:

In addition to medical intervention, lifestyle modifications and self, care practices can play a crucial role in managing sinusitis. Consider incorporating the following into your routine:

Healthy diet: Adopting a balanced diet rich in fruits, vegetables, whole grains, and lean proteins can support your immune system and overall health. Certain nutrients, such as vitamin C and antioxidants, may help reduce inflammation.

Hydration: Drink plenty of water throughout the day to keep your body hydrated and promote healthy mucus production. Proper hydration can help thin mucus and facilitate its removal from the sinuses.

Finding a Healthcare Provider

Finding a Healthcare Provider: Your Guide to Effective Sinusitis Care

When it comes to managing sinusitis, having a reliable and experienced healthcare provider is essential. Whether you're seeking diagnosis, treatment, or ongoing management, finding the right healthcare professional can make a significant difference in your sinusitis journey. Below we will explore the steps involved in finding a healthcare provider who specializes in sinusitis, ensuring that you receive the best care and support for your condition.

Start with Your Primary Care Physician:

Your primary care physician (PCP) is often the first healthcare professional you consult when experiencing sinusitis symptoms. They play a crucial role in evaluating your condition, providing initial treatment, and guiding you through the next steps. Here's what you can do:

Schedule an appointment: Reach out to your PCP and schedule an appointment to discuss your symptoms. Be prepared to provide a detailed description of your symptoms, their duration, and any previous treatments you have tried.

Communicate openly: During the appointment, communicate your concerns, any limitations sinusitis is causing in your daily life, and your goals for treatment. Be honest about your symptoms, including their impact on your physical and emotional well, being.

Seek referrals: If your PCP determines that your condition requires further evaluation or specialized care, they can provide you with referrals to healthcare providers who specialize in sinusitis, such as an ear, nose, and throat (ENT) specialist or an allergist.

Research and Gather Information:

Once you have a referral or decide to seek specialized care independently, conducting thorough research can help you make an informed decision. Consider the following steps:

Check credentials and expertise: Look for healthcare providers who specialize in sinusitis or related conditions. Review their qualifications, certifications, and years of experience. Ensure they have a strong background in diagnosing and treating sinusitis.

Read patient reviews and testimonials: Online platforms and websites often feature patient reviews and testimonials. Pay attention to others' experiences with the healthcare provider, their satisfaction with the treatment received, and the provider's communication style and bedside manner.

Look for affiliations with reputable organizations: Check if the healthcare provider is affiliated with professional organizations, such as the American Academy of Otolaryngology, Head and Neck Surgery (AAO, HNS). Membership in such organizations indicates a commitment to upholding high standards of care.

Consider Specialty Providers:

Sinusitis can be complex, and in some cases, it may be necessary to consult with specialists who have specific expertise in diagnosing and treating sinus conditions. Consider the following specialty providers:

Ear, Nose, and Throat (ENT) specialists: These physicians focus on conditions affecting the ears, nose, and throat. ENT specialists have extensive knowledge and experience in diagnosing and treating sinusitis, including more severe or chronic cases that may require surgical intervention.

Allergists: If your sinusitis is related to allergies, an allergist can help identify specific allergens that may be triggering your symptoms. They can conduct allergy testing, develop personalized treatment plans, and provide guidance on managing allergies to prevent sinusitis flare, ups.

Evaluate Communication and Compatibility:

When visiting potential healthcare providers, pay attention to their communication style and how comfortable you feel interacting with them. Effective communication and a positive doctor, patient relationship are crucial for successful treatment. Consider the following factors:

Active listening: The healthcare provider should actively listen to your concerns, ask relevant questions, and demonstrate empathy and understanding.

Clear communication: The provider should be able to explain your condition, treatment options, and expected outcomes in clear and understandable terms. They should encourage your involvement in decision, making.

Support Groups

Support Groups: Connecting with Others on the Sinusitis Journey

Living with sinusitis can be challenging, both physically and emotionally. The symptoms, treatment options, and daily management can sometimes feel overwhelming. In such times, having a support system can make a significant difference in coping with the condition. Support groups provide a platform for individuals with sinusitis to connect, share experiences, exchange information, and offer emotional support. Below we will explore the benefits of support groups and how they can enhance the well, being of those living with sinusitis.

Shared Experiences:

One of the most valuable aspects of support groups is the opportunity to connect with others who are facing similar challenges. Sharing experiences with individuals who truly understand the impact of sinusitis can be comforting and validating. It creates a sense of community and reduces feelings of isolation. Through these interactions, you may gain insights, learn coping strategies, and develop a sense of empowerment in managing your condition.

Emotional Support:

Dealing with a chronic condition like sinusitis can take a toll on your emotional well, being. Support groups offer a safe space where you can openly express your feelings, fears, and frustrations. Participants can empathize with your struggles and provide encouragement, empathy, and understanding. Sharing emotional burdens within a supportive environment can alleviate stress, anxiety, and depression often associated with chronic illnesses.

Information and Education:

Support groups serve as a valuable source of information and education. Participants can share knowledge about the latest treatment options, home remedies, and self, care strategies they have found effective in managing their sinusitis. These discussions can provide insights into alternative therapies, dietary changes, and lifestyle modifications that may complement medical treatments. However, it's important to remember that support groups are not a substitute for professional medical advice, and any new treatments or approaches should be discussed with your healthcare provider.

Practical Tips and Advice:

Support groups offer a wealth of practical tips and advice from individuals who have firsthand experience with sinusitis. Participants may share techniques for symptom relief, such as effective ways to manage congestion, headaches, or facial pain. They may also offer suggestions on navigating healthcare systems, finding the right healthcare providers, or dealing with insurance, related challenges. The shared wisdom and collective knowledge within the group can be invaluable in improving your day, to, day management of sinusitis.

Motivation and Empowerment:

Being part of a support group can provide motivation and inspiration on your sinusitis journey. Witnessing the resilience and determination of others can ignite a sense of hope and optimism. Participants often celebrate milestones, share success stories, and encourage each other to stay proactive in managing their condition. This positive reinforcement can boost your confidence and empower you to take an active role in your own health and well, being.

Online Support Groups:

In addition to in, person support groups, online communities have become increasingly popular and accessible. Online support groups provide convenience, especially for those who may have difficulty attending physical meetings due to geographic limitations or health constraints. These virtual communities offer a platform for individuals to connect, engage in discussions, and receive support from the comfort of their own homes. Online support groups may exist on social media platforms, dedicated websites, or specialized forums.

Finding Support Groups:

Finding a support group for sinusitis may require some research and exploration. Here are some ways to locate support groups:

Online searches: Use search engines to look for support groups specifically focused on sinusitis or related conditions. Include keywords like "sinusitis support group" or "chronic sinusitis community."

Medical professionals: Consult with your healthcare provider, such as your primary care physician, ENT specialist, or allergist, for recommendations on local support groups or online communities.

Online Resources

Online Resources: A Wealth of Information and Support for Sinusitis

In today's digital age, the internet has become a vast repository of information on various health topics, including sinusitis. Whether you're seeking in, depth medical knowledge, self, help tips, or a supportive community, online resources can provide a wealth of information and support for individuals living with sinusitis. Below we will explore the benefits and diverse offerings of online resources in relation to sinusitis.

Educational Websites and Articles:

Numerous reputable websites and online articles offer comprehensive information on sinusitis. These resources provide a deep dive into the causes, symptoms, diagnosis, and treatment options for sinusitis. They often include detailed explanations of medical concepts, anatomy, and physiology related to the condition. Educational websites may be run by medical institutions, professional organizations, or trusted health platforms, ensuring reliable and evidence, based information.

Medical Journals and Research Papers:

For those interested in delving into the latest scientific advancements and research on sinusitis, online medical journals and research databases are invaluable resources. These platforms provide access to peer, reviewed studies, clinical trials, and scholarly articles written by experts in the field. By exploring scientific literature, individuals can stay updated on emerging treatment modalities, novel therapies, and diagnostic techniques.

Online Medical Forums and Communities:

Online medical forums and communities offer a platform for individuals to connect, share experiences, and seek advice from others who are going through similar journeys. These platforms foster peer, to, peer support, allowing individuals to ask questions, share concerns, and provide support to one another. Active participation in online discussions can provide emotional support, practical tips, and a sense of belonging.

Social Media Groups and Pages:

Social media platforms have become powerful tools for disseminating health, related information and creating online communities. Various social media groups and pages are dedicated to sinusitis, where individuals can join discussions, follow informative posts, and connect with others facing similar challenges. These groups often provide a mixture of educational content, personal anecdotes, and updates on research and treatment advancements.

Online Symptom Checkers:

In cases where individuals experience symptoms but are unsure if they are related to sinusitis or another condition, online symptom checkers can be useful. These tools allow users to enter their symptoms and receive possible explanations and recommendations. While online symptom checkers can provide a general idea of potential causes, it's important to consult with a healthcare professional for an accurate diagnosis.

Telemedicine and Virtual Consultations:

The rise of telemedicine has revolutionized access to healthcare services, especially for individuals with limited mobility or those living in remote areas. Virtual consultations with healthcare providers allow individuals to seek medical advice, discuss symptoms, and receive treatment recommendations without the need for in, person visits. Telemedicine is particularly beneficial for follow, up appointments, medication refills, and routine check, ins with healthcare professionals.

Online Treatment and Self, Care Resources:

Online resources offer a plethora of self, care strategies and treatment recommendations for sinusitis. From home remedies and natural therapies to lifestyle modifications and dietary suggestions, individuals can find a wide range of approaches to complement medical treatments. However, it's crucial to exercise caution and consult with a healthcare professional before implementing any new treatment regimen.

Video Tutorials and Demonstrations:

Visual learning can be an effective way to understand sinusitis management techniques. Online platforms provide video tutorials and demonstrations of various self, care practices, such as nasal irrigation techniques, steam inhalation, or facial massage. These videos offer step, by, step guidance, ensuring individuals can perform these activities correctly and safely.

Webinars and Online Seminars:

Webinars and online seminars conducted by medical professionals and experts in the field of sinusitis provide an opportunity to learn from the comfort of one's own home.

Chapter Twenty

Sinusitis and the Immune System

Sinusitis and the Immune System: Understanding the Connection

The immune system is a complex network of cells, tissues, and organs that play a vital role in defending the body against harmful pathogens and maintaining overall health. When it comes to sinusitis, an inflammatory condition affecting the sinuses, the immune system plays a crucial role in both its development and resolution. Below we will explore the connection between sinusitis and the immune system, shedding light on the intricate mechanisms involved.

The immune response to sinusitis begins with the recognition of pathogens or allergens that have invaded the sinuses. The sinuses are hollow cavities located within the facial bones, and they are lined with mucous membranes. These membranes produce mucus, which helps to trap and remove foreign particles, bacteria, and viruses. However, when the sinuses become inflamed, either due to infection or allergic reactions, the immune response is triggered.

Inflammatory Response:

When the immune system detects the presence of pathogens or allergens in the sinuses, it initiates an inflammatory response. This response involves the release of various chemicals, such as histamines, leukotrienes, and cytokines, which cause the blood vessels in the sinuses to dilate and become more permeable. This increased blood flow and permeability help deliver immune cells to the affected area to combat the infection or allergen.

Immune Cell Activation:

During sinusitis, immune cells, including neutrophils, macrophages, and lymphocytes, are mobilized to the sinuses to fight off the invading pathogens or allergens. Neutrophils are the first line of defense and are responsible for engulfing and destroying bacteria. Macrophages, on the other hand, are scavenger cells that engulf and break down pathogens and cellular debris. Lymphocytes, a type of white blood cell, play a key role in the adaptive immune response by recognizing and targeting specific pathogens.

Allergic Response:

In some cases, sinusitis is triggered by an allergic reaction to environmental allergens such as pollen, dust mites, or pet dander. When these allergens enter the sinuses, the immune system overreacts, causing an allergic response. In allergic sinusitis, the immune system releases antibodies, such as immunoglobulin E (IgE), in response to the allergen. These antibodies bind to mast cells, triggering the release of histamine and other chemicals that cause inflammation and allergic symptoms.

Immune System Dysfunction:

In certain individuals, the immune system may not function optimally, leading to an increased susceptibility to sinusitis. Immunodeficiency disorders, such as primary immunodeficiency diseases or acquired immunodeficiency syndrome (AIDS), weaken the immune system's ability to fight off infections. As a result, individuals with immunodeficiency are more prone to recurrent or chronic sinusitis.

On the other hand, an overactive immune system can also contribute to sinusitis. Autoimmune disorders, such as systemic lupus erythematosus or Wegener's granulomatosis, can cause inflammation in the sinuses and nasal passages, leading to chronic sinusitis. In these cases, the immune system mistakenly attacks healthy tissues in the sinuses, perpetuating the inflammatory response.

Immune System Modulation:

Given the critical role of the immune system in sinusitis, various treatment approaches aim to modulate or regulate immune responses. Immunotherapy, for example, involves the administration of allergen extracts to desensitize the immune system and reduce allergic reactions. This approach is particularly beneficial for individuals with allergic sinusitis. Immunomodulatory medications, such as corticosteroids, can also be prescribed to suppress the immune response and reduce inflammation in cases of chronic or severe sinusitis.

Role of the Immune System in Sinusitis

The Role of the Immune System in Sinusitis: A Key Player in Defense

Sinusitis is a common condition characterized by the inflammation and swelling of the sinuses, which are hollow cavities in the skull connected to the nasal passages. While various factors can contribute to the development of sinusitis, the immune system plays a critical role in both the onset and resolution of this condition. Below we will explore the intricate relationship between sinusitis and the immune system, highlighting its important role in defending the body against pathogens and maintaining sinus health.

When the sinuses become inflamed due to infection, allergies, or other triggers, the immune system springs into action to combat the threat. Let's delve into the mechanisms involved:

Recognizing the Threat:

The immune system's first task is to recognize the presence of pathogens, allergens, or irritants in the sinuses. This recognition occurs through specialized cells, such as macrophages and dendritic cells, which patrol the sinuses and sample the environment for any foreign invaders. These cells act as sentinels, detecting the presence of bacteria, viruses, or allergens and initiating an immune response.

Initiating the Inflammatory Response:

Upon detection of a threat, the immune system triggers an inflammatory response to eliminate the invading pathogens or clear the allergens. The initial step is the release of chemical signals, such as histamines and cytokines, which induce vasodilation and increase the permeability of blood vessels in the sinuses. This allows immune cells to reach the site of infection or allergen exposure more efficiently.

Mobilizing Immune Cells:

The immune system dispatches a variety of immune cells to the sinuses to eliminate the threat. Neutrophils, a type of white blood cell, are among the first responders. They quickly migrate to the infected or inflamed sinuses, where they engulf and destroy bacteria or other foreign particles. Macrophages, another type of immune cell, play a vital role in clearing away dead cells, debris, and pathogens, ensuring a clean and healthy sinus environment. Lymphocytes, including T cells and B cells, coordinate the adaptive immune response and produce specific antibodies to neutralize the invading pathogens.

Antibody Production:

When confronted with bacteria or viruses, the immune system produces specific antibodies that bind to these pathogens and mark them for destruction. In sinusitis, this antibody production is crucial for effectively eliminating the infecting microbes. Immunoglobulin A (IgA), in particular, plays a key role in mucosal immunity, protecting the sinus membranes from infection.

Impact of Allergic Reactions:

In allergic sinusitis, the immune system reacts excessively to harmless substances, such as pollen or dust mites, triggering an allergic response. This hypersensitivity is due to the production of Immunoglobulin E (IgE) antibodies, which recognize and bind to allergens. The binding of IgE to allergens activates mast cells, leading to the release of inflammatory substances like histamines. This causes the characteristic symptoms of allergic sinusitis, including nasal congestion, sneezing, and watery eyes.

Chronic Inflammation:

In some cases, the immune response in sinusitis becomes dysregulated, leading to chronic inflammation. Chronic sinusitis occurs when the immune system fails to completely eradicate the infection or when there is an ongoing immune response to persistent irritants or allergens. The prolonged inflammation can damage the sinus tissues and impede proper drainage, creating an ideal environment for bacteria to thrive and causing recurrent or chronic sinusitis.

Strengthening the Immune System

Strengthening the Immune System: Boosting Your Defenses Against Sinusitis

The immune system is a remarkable network of cells, tissues, and organs that works tirelessly to protect our bodies from harmful invaders. When it comes to sinusitis, a condition characterized by the inflammation of the sinuses, having a strong immune system is essential in preventing and fighting off infections. Below we will explore various strategies to strengthen the immune system and reduce the risk of sinusitis. By incorporating these practices into your lifestyle, you can enhance your body's natural defenses and promote sinus health.

Balanced Diet:

A nutritious diet is crucial for supporting a healthy immune system. Including a variety of fruits, vegetables, whole grains, lean proteins, and healthy fats provides the necessary vitamins, minerals, and antioxidants to optimize immune function. Vitamin C, found in citrus fruits and leafy greens, is known for its immune, boosting properties. Zinc, present in foods like nuts, seeds, and legumes, also plays a vital role in immune system function. Additionally, consuming probiotic, rich foods, such as yogurt and fermented vegetables, can promote a healthy balance of gut bacteria, which is closely linked to immune health.

Regular Exercise:

Engaging in regular physical activity offers numerous benefits, including immune system enhancement. Exercise increases blood circulation, promoting the efficient delivery of immune cells throughout the body. It also reduces stress hormones, which can suppress immune function. Aim for at least 150 minutes of moderate, intensity exercise per week, such as brisk walking, jogging, or cycling, to reap the immune, boosting benefits.

Quality Sleep:

Adequate sleep is vital for a well, functioning immune system. During sleep, the body produces and releases cytokines, proteins that regulate immune responses. Insufficient sleep can disrupt the production of these cytokines, weakening the immune response and increasing susceptibility to infections. Aim for 7, 8 hours of quality sleep each night to support optimal immune function and reduce the risk of sinusitis.

Stress Management:

Chronic stress can take a toll on the immune system, making the body more susceptible to infections. Finding effective stress management techniques, such as meditation, deep breathing exercises, or engaging in hobbies, can help reduce stress levels and promote immune system resilience. Additionally, seeking support from friends, family, or a therapist can provide valuable emotional and psychological support during challenging times.

Hydration:

Proper hydration is essential for maintaining optimal immune function. Water helps flush out toxins, supports the production of lymph, and keeps mucous membranes moist, which is particularly beneficial for sinus health. Aim to drink an adequate amount of water each day, and limit the consumption of dehydrating beverages, such as caffeinated or sugary drinks.

Avoid Smoking and Limit Alcohol Consumption:

Smoking damages the respiratory system, impairs ciliary function (tiny hair, like structures that help clear mucus and debris), and weakens the immune response, making individuals more susceptible to sinus infections. Quitting smoking or avoiding exposure to secondhand smoke is crucial for sinus health. Similarly, excessive alcohol consumption can suppress immune function and disrupt sleep patterns. Limit alcohol intake and drink in moderation to support a strong immune system.

Regular Handwashing:

Proper hand hygiene is a simple yet effective practice to prevent the spread of infections. Wash your hands with soap and water for at least 20 seconds, especially before eating, after using the bathroom, or after being in public spaces. If soap and water are not available, use an alcohol, based hand sanitizer.

Vaccinations:

Keeping up to date with vaccinations is an important aspect of maintaining a robust immune system. Immunizations protect against various infectious diseases, including those that can lead to sinusitis, such as the flu.

Autoimmunity and Sinusitis

Autoimmunity and Sinusitis: Understanding the Connection

Sinusitis is a common condition characterized by inflammation of the sinus cavities, causing symptoms such as nasal congestion, facial pain, and sinus pressure. While sinusitis is often attributed to infections or allergies, another factor that can contribute to its development is autoimmunity. Autoimmunity occurs when the immune system mistakenly attacks healthy cells and tissues in the body. Below we will explore the link between autoimmunity and sinusitis, shedding light on how an overactive immune response can play a role in the development and progression of sinusitis.

Autoimmune diseases are a group of disorders in which the immune system mistakenly identifies normal cells as foreign invaders and launches an immune response against them. This immune dysregulation can lead to chronic inflammation and tissue damage. Several autoimmune conditions have been associated with an increased risk of sinusitis, including:

Rheumatoid Arthritis (RA): RA is a chronic autoimmune disease that primarily affects the joints. However, it can also cause inflammation in other parts of the body, including the sinuses. The persistent inflammation in RA can disrupt the normal function of the sinuses, leading to chronic sinusitis.

Systemic Lupus Erythematosus (SLE): SLE is a systemic autoimmune disease that can affect multiple organs and tissues. In some individuals with SLE, the immune system may attack the sinuses, leading to recurrent sinus infections and chronic sinusitis.

Granulomatosis with Polyangiitis (GPA): GPA is a rare autoimmune disorder characterized by inflammation of blood vessels. The inflammation can extend to the sinuses, resulting in chronic sinusitis, nasal crusting, and nasal ulcers.

Sjögren's Syndrome: Sjögren's syndrome is an autoimmune disease that primarily affects the moisture, producing glands, leading to dry eyes and dry mouth. It can also cause inflammation in the sinuses, contributing to the development of sinusitis.

Autoimmune, related sinusitis often presents with distinct characteristics compared to other forms of sinusitis. It tends to be chronic and recurrent, with symptoms that persist for an extended period. Additionally, autoimmune, related sinusitis may be associated with other systemic symptoms related to the underlying autoimmune condition, such as joint pain, fatigue, or skin rashes.

The exact mechanisms by which autoimmunity contributes to sinusitis are not fully understood. However, several hypotheses have been proposed. One theory suggests that autoantibodies, which are produced by the immune system in autoimmune diseases, can target the sinus tissues and trigger inflammation. Another theory suggests that the chronic inflammation caused by autoimmunity weakens the sinus tissues, making them more susceptible to infections.

Managing sinusitis in individuals with autoimmune diseases requires a comprehensive approach that addresses both the autoimmune condition and the sinusitis symptoms. Treatment strategies may include:

Immunosuppressive Medications: In autoimmune, related sinusitis, medications that suppress the immune system may be prescribed to reduce inflammation and control the autoimmune response. These medications can help alleviate sinusitis symptoms and prevent further damage to the sinuses.

Nasal Irrigation: Regular nasal irrigation with saline solution can help clear the sinuses, reduce inflammation, and alleviate symptoms. This simple and effective technique can be performed using a neti pot, nasal spray, or nasal irrigator.

Symptom Management: Over, the, counter medications, such as decongestants and pain relievers, may be recommended to manage symptoms like nasal congestion, facial pain, and headache. However, it is important to consult with a healthcare professional before starting any new medications, especially for individuals with autoimmune conditions who may be taking other medications.

Collaboration with Specialists: Individuals with autoimmune, related sinusitis may benefit from collaborating with a team of healthcare providers.

Chapter Twenty-One

The Role of Exercise in Sinus Health

Sinusitis is a condition characterized by inflammation of the sinus cavities, leading to symptoms such as nasal congestion, facial pain, and sinus pressure. While medications and other treatments are commonly used to manage sinusitis, the role of exercise in sinus health is often overlooked. Engaging in regular physical activity can have a positive impact on sinus health, helping to alleviate symptoms, reduce the frequency of sinus infections, and promote overall well, being. Below we will explore the benefits of exercise for sinus health and discuss various types of exercises that can be beneficial for individuals with sinusitis.

Exercise offers a range of benefits for sinus health. Firstly, it promotes circulation and blood flow throughout the body, including the sinus cavities. This increased blood flow helps to deliver oxygen and nutrients to the sinus tissues, supporting their optimal function and aiding in the clearance of mucus and debris. Improved circulation also enhances the body's immune response, helping to prevent and fight off infections.

Regular exercise can also help manage sinusitis symptoms by reducing nasal congestion. When we engage in physical activity, our breathing rate increases, and deeper inhalations and exhalations occur. This can help clear the nasal passages, allowing for better airflow and reducing congestion. Additionally, exercise promotes the release of endorphins, natural pain, relieving chemicals that can help alleviate facial pain and headaches associated with sinusitis.

Certain types of exercises are particularly beneficial for sinus health. Aerobic exercises, such as brisk walking, jogging, cycling, or swimming, are excellent choices. These activities increase heart rate and respiratory rate, promoting deep breathing and enhanced blood flow. They also help strengthen the cardiovascular system, which supports overall health and immune function.

Yoga and deep breathing exercises are also beneficial for sinus health. These practices focus on deep, controlled breathing, which can help clear the nasal passages and promote relaxation. Specific yoga poses, such as the forward fold or downward, facing dog, can help drain the sinuses by promoting drainage and relieving congestion.

It's important to note that individuals with sinusitis should consider the following tips when incorporating exercise into their routine:

Start Slowly: If you are new to exercise or have been inactive for a while, it's important to start slowly and gradually increase intensity and duration. This allows your body to adapt and minimize the risk of overexertion or worsening sinus symptoms.

Stay Hydrated: Proper hydration is crucial for overall health and sinus function. Drinking an adequate amount of water before, during, and after exercise helps maintain healthy mucus production and prevents dehydration, which can exacerbate sinusitis symptoms.

Consider Environmental Factors: If you have sinusitis triggered by allergies or environmental irritants, it's essential to be mindful of the exercise environment. Avoid exercising outdoors during high pollen or pollution levels, and consider wearing a mask or exercising indoors on days when the air quality is poor.

Manage Post, Exercise Nasal Symptoms: Some individuals may experience increased nasal congestion or post, exercise rhinitis. To manage these symptoms, try rinsing your nasal passages with saline solution after exercise or using a nasal spray to reduce inflammation.

Incorporating regular exercise into your routine not only benefits sinus health but also promotes overall well, being. It can help reduce stress, improve sleep quality, boost energy levels, and enhance mood. However, it's important to listen to your body and modify or discontinue exercise if it exacerbates sinus symptoms or causes discomfort.

Benefits of Exercise for Sinus Health

Sinusitis is a common condition characterized by inflammation of the sinus cavities, leading to symptoms such as nasal congestion, facial pain, and pressure. While medication and other treatments are often used to manage sinusitis, the role of exercise in promoting sinus health is often overlooked. Engaging in regular physical activity can have numerous benefits for individuals with sinusitis, including improved sinus drainage, reduced congestion, and enhanced overall well, being. Below we will explore the benefits of exercise for sinus health and discuss how incorporating physical activity into your routine can help alleviate sinusitis symptoms.

Improved Sinus Drainage: One of the key benefits of exercise for sinus health is improved sinus drainage. When we engage in physical activity, such as brisk walking, jogging, or cycling, our breathing rate increases, and deeper breaths are taken. This helps to stimulate the movement of mucus within the sinus cavities, promoting drainage and reducing congestion. Enhanced sinus drainage allows for better airflow, alleviating symptoms and promoting sinus health.

Strengthened Immune System: Regular exercise has been shown to boost immune function, which is essential for preventing and fighting off infections, including sinus infections. Exercise increases blood flow and circulation throughout the body, including the sinuses, allowing immune cells to reach infected areas more effectively. Additionally, exercise promotes the production of antibodies and enhances the activity of immune cells, helping to defend against pathogens and reduce the risk of sinusitis.

Reduced Inflammation: Sinusitis is often associated with inflammation in the sinus cavities. Exercise has been shown to have anti, inflammatory effects, helping to reduce overall inflammation in the body, including the sinuses. By reducing inflammation, exercise can alleviate symptoms such as facial pain and pressure, and contribute to improved sinus health.

Enhanced Respiratory Health: Regular physical activity improves respiratory function and lung capacity. This can be particularly beneficial for individuals with sinusitis, as it helps to optimize breathing and reduce nasal congestion. Improved respiratory health allows for better oxygen exchange and helps to clear the nasal passages, making breathing easier and reducing sinusitis symptoms.

Stress Reduction: Chronic sinusitis can have a significant impact on an individual's quality of life and overall well, being. Exercise is known to reduce stress levels and promote the release of endorphins, which are natural mood enhancers. By incorporating exercise into your routine, you can effectively manage stress and improve your mental well, being, which in turn can have a positive impact on your sinus health.

Weight Management: Maintaining a healthy weight is important for sinus health, as excess weight can contribute to increased pressure in the sinuses and exacerbate symptoms. Regular exercise, combined with a balanced diet, can help manage weight and reduce the burden on the sinuses, leading to improved overall sinus health.

Improved Sleep Quality: Sinusitis can often disrupt sleep due to symptoms such as nasal congestion and facial pain. Regular exercise has been shown to improve sleep quality and promote better sleep patterns. By getting an adequate amount of restful sleep, individuals with sinusitis can experience reduced symptoms and improved overall well, being.

It's important to note that individuals with sinusitis should consider the following tips when incorporating exercise into their routine:

Start slowly and gradually increase intensity and duration to avoid overexertion and worsening of symptoms.

Stay hydrated by drinking enough water before, during, and after exercise to maintain healthy mucus production and prevent dehydration.

Be mindful of environmental factors that may trigger sinusitis symptoms, such as allergens or irritants, and adjust exercise locations or times accordingly.

Consider consulting with a healthcare professional or sinus specialist to ensure that exercise is safe and appropriate for your specific condition.

Best Exercises for Sinusitis

The Best Exercises for Sinusitis: Promoting Sinus Health through Physical Activity

Sinusitis, characterized by inflammation and congestion in the sinus cavities, can cause discomfort and affect daily life. While medication and other treatments are commonly used to manage sinusitis, incorporating specific exercises into your routine can provide additional relief and promote sinus health. Below we will explore the best exercises for sinusitis, focusing on activities that can help improve sinus drainage, alleviate congestion, and enhance overall well, being.

Aerobic Exercises: Aerobic exercises, also known as cardiovascular exercises, are great for promoting sinus health. Activities like brisk walking, jogging, cycling, swimming, and dancing increase heart rate and breathing, improving blood circulation and promoting sinus drainage. These exercises also help to strengthen the respiratory system, enhance lung capacity, and reduce congestion.

Yoga: Yoga is a gentle and effective exercise option for individuals with sinusitis. Certain yoga poses can help open up the chest and nasal passages, facilitating better airflow and sinus drainage. Poses like the downward, facing dog, cat, cow, bridge pose, and supported fish pose can promote relaxation, reduce facial pressure, and improve sinus health. Additionally, practicing deep breathing exercises in yoga can further enhance respiratory function.

Pilates: Pilates is a low, impact exercise method that focuses on strengthening the core muscles, improving posture, and enhancing overall body awareness. By targeting the core muscles and promoting proper alignment, Pilates exercises can alleviate tension and strain in the neck, shoulders, and upper back, which are commonly associated with sinusitis. Improved posture can also help facilitate better breathing and sinus drainage.

Tai Chi: Tai Chi is a gentle, slow, moving martial art that combines fluid movements, deep breathing, and mindfulness. Regular practice of Tai Chi can help improve circulation, reduce stress, and enhance overall well, being. The slow, controlled movements of Tai Chi can promote relaxation, relieve tension in the neck and shoulders, and improve sinus drainage.

Facial Exercises: Specific facial exercises can help relieve sinus pressure and tension. These exercises involve gentle movements and massages that stimulate the facial muscles, promote circulation, and alleviate congestion. One example is the sinus pressure point massage, where gentle pressure is applied to specific points around the nose, cheeks, and forehead to relieve sinus pressure and improve drainage. Consult with a healthcare professional or physical therapist for guidance on facial exercises specific to sinusitis.

Breathing Exercises: Deep breathing exercises can be particularly beneficial for individuals with sinusitis. Techniques like diaphragmatic breathing and alternate nostril breathing help expand the lungs, promote relaxation, and enhance sinus drainage. These exercises can be done anywhere and at any time, providing immediate relief from congestion and promoting overall sinus health.

Low, Impact Strength Training: Engaging in low, impact strength training exercises, such as using resistance bands or light weights, can help strengthen the muscles supporting the upper body, including the neck, shoulders, and back. By improving muscle tone and stability, these exercises can reduce strain on the sinuses and improve posture, leading to better breathing and reduced sinusitis symptoms.

When engaging in exercise for sinusitis, it is essential to keep the following tips in mind:

Start slowly and gradually increase the intensity and duration of your workouts to avoid overexertion and exacerbation of symptoms.

Stay hydrated by drinking enough water before, during, and after exercise to maintain healthy mucus production and prevent dehydration.

Pay attention to your body and modify or stop exercises that worsen your sinusitis symptoms.

Consider working with a qualified fitness professional or physical therapist who can provide guidance and tailor exercises to your specific needs and limitations.

Precautions While Exercising

Precautions While Exercising: Safely Managing Sinusitis Symptoms during Physical Activity

Regular exercise is crucial for maintaining overall health and well, being. However, when dealing with sinusitis, it's important to take certain precautions to ensure that physical activity does not exacerbate symptoms or cause discomfort. Below we will discuss the precautions to consider while exercising with sinusitis, helping you manage your condition effectively and safely.

Consult with Your Healthcare Provider: Before starting any exercise program, it's essential to consult with your healthcare provider, especially if you have severe or chronic sinusitis. They can provide personalized guidance based on your specific condition, medical history, and current symptoms. Your healthcare provider may recommend modifications to your exercise routine or suggest alternative activities that are better suited to your needs.

Choose the Right Time and Environment: When planning your exercise routine, consider the time of day and the environment in which you will be exercising. For some individuals with sinusitis, outdoor activities during certain times of the year or in specific weather conditions may trigger symptoms. Pollen, pollutants, and cold air can worsen congestion and sinus pressure. If you are sensitive to these factors, opt for indoor exercises or choose outdoor activities during periods when allergens or irritants are less prevalent.

Warm, Up and Cool, Down: Prior to engaging in any physical activity, it's important to warm up your body. A proper warm, up helps increase blood flow, prepare your muscles, and reduce the risk of injury. Incorporate gentle exercises such as stretching or light cardio to gradually increase your heart rate and loosen up your muscles. Similarly, after your workout, cool down with some light stretching to promote muscle recovery and prevent stiffness.

Pay Attention to Breathing: Sinusitis can affect nasal airflow and make breathing through the nose difficult. If nasal congestion is present, focus on breathing through your mouth during exercise. This can help you maintain proper oxygen intake and minimize discomfort. Additionally, practicing proper breathing techniques, such as diaphragmatic breathing or pursed lip breathing, can enhance lung capacity and reduce strain on the respiratory system.

Modify Intensity and Duration: Sinusitis symptoms can vary from person to person and from day to day. It's important to listen to your body and adjust the intensity and duration of your workouts accordingly. If you're experiencing severe symptoms or a flare, up, it may be necessary to reduce the intensity or take a break from exercise until you feel better. Gradually increase the intensity and duration of your workouts as your symptoms improve.

Stay Hydrated: Hydration is important for overall health and can also help manage sinusitis symptoms. Drink plenty of water before, during, and after exercise to stay hydrated. Proper hydration helps maintain healthy mucus production, which facilitates better sinus drainage. Avoid excessive caffeine and alcohol intake, as they can contribute to dehydration and worsen symptoms.

Be Mindful of Environmental Irritants: Certain environments or activities can expose you to irritants that may trigger or worsen sinusitis symptoms. Avoid smoke, strong odors, chemicals, and other airborne irritants. If you're exercising indoors, ensure good ventilation to minimize exposure to allergens or irritants. If you're exercising outdoors, consider wearing a mask to filter out particles and reduce exposure to allergens or pollutants.

Listen to Your Body: It's crucial to pay attention to your body's signals while exercising with sinusitis. If you experience increased pain, pressure, dizziness, or severe discomfort, it's important to stop and rest. Pushing through excessive discomfort can potentially worsen your symptoms and delay your recovery. Modify or change exercises as needed to minimize stress on your sinuses and seek medical attention if necessary.

Chapter Twenty-Two

Complementary and Alternative Treatments

Complementary and Alternative Treatments for Sinusitis: Exploring Additional Options for Relief

Sinusitis, also known as a sinus infection, can cause significant discomfort and affect daily life. While conventional medical treatments such as medications and surgery are commonly used, some individuals seek alternative approaches to manage their symptoms. Complementary and alternative treatments offer additional options for relief and may be used in conjunction with traditional treatments. Below we will explore various complementary and alternative treatments for sinusitis, providing an overview of their benefits, effectiveness, and considerations.

Nasal Irrigation: Nasal irrigation, also known as nasal rinsing or saline irrigation, involves flushing the nasal passages with a saline solution. This technique helps moisturize the nasal passages, reduce inflammation, and remove mucus and allergens. It can be done using a neti pot, nasal spray, or nasal irrigation bottle. Nasal irrigation is generally safe and well, tolerated, but it's important to use sterile saline solutions and follow proper hygiene practices to prevent infections.

Steam Inhalation: Steam inhalation involves breathing in warm, moist air to help alleviate congestion and promote sinus drainage. It can be done by leaning over a bowl of hot water with a towel over the head or using a steam inhaler. The warm steam helps soothe the nasal passages, loosen mucus, and relieve sinus pressure. Adding essential oils such as eucalyptus or peppermint to the steam can provide additional benefits. However, caution should be exercised when using steam inhalation to avoid burns or excessive heat exposure.

Herbal Remedies: Certain herbal remedies may offer relief from sinusitis symptoms. Eucalyptus, for example, is known for its decongestant and anti, inflammatory properties. It can be used in the form of essential oil, steam inhalation, or topical ointments. Other herbs such as chamomile, ginger, and turmeric may also have anti, inflammatory and immune, boosting effects. While herbal remedies can be helpful, it's important to consult with a healthcare provider or herbalist for appropriate dosages and potential interactions with medications.

Acupuncture: Acupuncture is a traditional Chinese medicine practice that involves the insertion of thin needles into specific points on the body. It is believed to help rebalance the body's energy flow and promote healing. Some studies suggest that acupuncture may be beneficial for sinusitis by reducing inflammation, relieving pain, and improving nasal airflow. However, more research is needed to establish its effectiveness. It's important to seek acupuncture treatment from a qualified practitioner to ensure safety and efficacy.

Acupressure: Acupressure involves applying pressure to specific points on the body using fingers, thumbs, or specialized tools. Similar to acupuncture, acupressure aims to stimulate specific energy pathways to alleviate symptoms. The facial sinus points, located around the nose, eyes, and forehead, can be targeted to relieve sinusitis symptoms. Applying gentle pressure to these points in a circular motion may help reduce congestion and promote sinus drainage. Acupressure can be done by oneself or with the assistance of a trained therapist.

Probiotics: Probiotics are beneficial bacteria that can help support a healthy immune system and maintain a balanced gut microbiome. Some research suggests that certain strains of probiotics, such as Lactobacillus and Bifidobacterium, may help reduce the frequency and severity of respiratory infections, including sinusitis. Probiotics can be consumed through fermented foods like yogurt, kefir, sauerkraut, or as supplements. However, more studies are needed to determine the specific strains and dosages that are effective for sinusitis.

Acupuncture and Sinusitis

Acupuncture and Sinusitis: Exploring the Potential Benefits of Traditional Chinese Medicine

Sinusitis, a condition characterized by inflammation of the sinus cavities, can cause significant discomfort and impact daily life. While conventional treatments such as medications and nasal irrigation are commonly used, some individuals seek alternative approaches to manage their symptoms. Acupuncture, a key component of traditional Chinese medicine, is one such alternative treatment that has gained popularity in recent years. Below we will explore the potential benefits of acupuncture in the context of sinusitis, examining its principles, effectiveness, and considerations.

Acupuncture is a practice that originated in ancient China and involves the insertion of thin needles into specific points on the body. According to traditional Chinese medicine, the body has a network of meridians or energy pathways through which Qi (pronounced "chee"), the vital life force, flows. Illness or discomfort is believed to occur when there is an imbalance or blockage in the flow of Qi. Acupuncture aims to restore balance and promote healing by stimulating specific acupuncture points along the meridians.

When it comes to sinusitis, acupuncture is thought to work by reducing inflammation, improving blood circulation, and promoting the body's natural healing processes. By targeting specific acupuncture points, the flow of Qi can be restored, helping to alleviate sinusitis symptoms. The acupuncture points commonly used for sinusitis are located on the face, head, and neck areas, corresponding to the sinuses and related structures.

Several studies have explored the effectiveness of acupuncture in managing sinusitis symptoms. A systematic review published in the American Journal of Rhinology & Allergy in 2015 analyzed multiple studies and found that acupuncture was associated with significant improvement in nasal symptoms, including congestion, sneezing, and nasal discharge. Another study published in the Journal of Alternative and Complementary Medicine in 2016 reported that acupuncture resulted in a reduction of sinusitis symptoms and an improvement in the quality of life of the participants.

It is believed that acupuncture can help regulate the immune response and modulate inflammatory processes, which are crucial factors in sinusitis. By stimulating acupuncture points, the body's natural defense mechanisms can be activated, promoting a balanced immune response and reducing inflammation in the sinuses. However, it's important to note that individual responses to acupuncture may vary, and more research is needed to fully understand its mechanisms and effectiveness for sinusitis.

When considering acupuncture for sinusitis, it's essential to consult a licensed and qualified acupuncturist. They will conduct a thorough assessment and develop an individualized treatment plan based on the specific symptoms and underlying causes of sinusitis. Acupuncture sessions typically involve the insertion of fine needles into designated points on the face, scalp, and body. The needles are usually left in place for a certain period, ranging from a few minutes to half an hour, while the individual lies comfortably.

Many people find acupuncture to be a relaxing and therapeutic experience. The needles used in acupuncture are very thin and generally cause minimal discomfort. Some individuals may experience a slight tingling or warmth around the insertion points. It's important to communicate any sensations or concerns with the acupuncturist during the treatment session.

It's worth noting that acupuncture is generally considered safe when performed by a trained professional using sterile needles. However, certain precautions should be taken into account. Individuals with bleeding disorders or those taking blood, thinning medications may need to avoid acupuncture or inform their healthcare provider before starting treatment. Additionally, pregnant women should consult their healthcare provider before undergoing acupuncture.

While acupuncture can provide relief for sinusitis symptoms, it is often used as a complementary therapy alongside conventional treatments. It's important to work collaboratively with a healthcare provider to develop a comprehensive treatment plan that may include medications, nasal irrigation, and lifestyle modifications.

Herbal Remedies

Herbal Remedies for Sinusitis: Exploring Natural Approaches to Relieve Symptoms

Sinusitis, a condition characterized by inflammation of the sinus cavities, can cause discomfort and disrupt daily life. While conventional treatments are commonly used to manage sinusitis, some individuals seek natural alternatives to alleviate their symptoms. Herbal remedies, derived from plants and botanical sources, have been used for centuries in traditional medicine systems around the world. Below we will explore the potential benefits of herbal remedies in the context of sinusitis, examining their effectiveness, common herbs used, and considerations for use.

Herbal remedies for sinusitis aim to alleviate symptoms, reduce inflammation, and support the body's natural healing processes. They can be used in various forms, including teas, tinctures, capsules, and topical applications. It's important to note that herbal remedies should not replace conventional medical treatment for sinusitis, but rather be used as complementary approaches.

One commonly used herb for sinusitis is Echinacea. Echinacea is believed to enhance the immune system and reduce inflammation. It is often used to support the body's defense against respiratory infections, including sinusitis. Studies have suggested that Echinacea may help reduce the severity and duration of upper respiratory tract infections, although more research is needed to confirm its specific effects on sinusitis.

Another popular herb used for sinusitis is Goldenseal. Goldenseal contains a compound called berberine, which has antimicrobial properties. It is believed to help fight bacterial and fungal infections, which can be contributing factors to sinusitis. However, it's important to note that Goldenseal should be used with caution and under the guidance of a healthcare professional, as it can interact with certain medications and may not be suitable for everyone.

Ginger is another herb that may offer relief for sinusitis symptoms. Ginger has anti, inflammatory properties and can help reduce nasal congestion and relieve headaches associated with sinusitis. It can be consumed as a tea or added to meals for its warming and soothing effects. Ginger is generally safe for most people, but individuals taking blood, thinning medications should consult their healthcare provider before using it.

Peppermint is a well, known herb that can provide relief for sinusitis symptoms. Its menthol content helps open up nasal passages, reduce congestion, and relieve headaches. Peppermint tea or inhaling the steam from peppermint, infused hot water can provide soothing effects. However, caution should be exercised for individuals with gastroesophageal reflux disease (GERD), as peppermint may worsen symptoms.

Another herb commonly used in traditional medicine for sinusitis is Stinging Nettle. Stinging Nettle has anti, inflammatory properties and may help reduce nasal congestion and allergic reactions that can contribute to sinusitis. It can be consumed as a tea or taken as a supplement. However, it's important to note that Stinging Nettle can interact with certain medications, such as blood thinners and diuretics, so it's advisable to consult a healthcare professional before use.

Steam inhalation with herbs such as Eucalyptus, Rosemary, or Thyme can also provide relief for sinusitis symptoms. Adding a few drops of essential oil from these herbs to hot water and inhaling the steam can help soothe nasal passages, reduce congestion, and promote sinus drainage. However, caution should be exercised when using essential oils, as they are highly concentrated and should be diluted properly before use.

When using herbal remedies for sinusitis, it's essential to consider potential allergies or sensitivities to certain herbs. Some individuals may have allergic reactions to specific plants or herbs, so it's important to start with small doses and observe any adverse reactions. Additionally, herbal remedies may interact with certain medications, so it's advisable to consult a healthcare professional, especially if you are taking prescription medications.

Aromatherapy

Aromatherapy for Sinusitis: Harnessing the Power of Essential Oils for Relief

Sinusitis, a condition characterized by inflammation of the sinus cavities, can cause discomfort and disrupt daily life. While conventional treatments are commonly used to manage sinusitis, some individuals seek alternative approaches to alleviate their symptoms. Aromatherapy, a holistic practice that utilizes the scents of essential oils derived from plants, has gained popularity as a natural remedy for various health conditions, including sinusitis. Below we will explore the potential benefits of aromatherapy in the context of sinusitis, examining its effectiveness, common essential oils used, and considerations for use.

Aromatherapy involves the use of essential oils, highly concentrated extracts from plants, to promote physical and psychological well, being. These oils are typically obtained through distillation or cold pressing methods and contain the aromatic compounds that give plants their distinctive scents. When inhaled or applied topically, essential oils can have a range of effects on the body and mind.

One of the primary benefits of aromatherapy for sinusitis is its ability to alleviate nasal congestion and promote sinus drainage. Essential oils such as Eucalyptus, Peppermint, and Tea Tree are known for their decongestant properties. Inhalation of these oils can help open up the nasal passages, reduce inflammation, and facilitate the release of mucus, providing relief from congestion and improving breathing.

Eucalyptus essential oil is widely used in aromatherapy for sinusitis due to its expectorant and antimicrobial properties. It helps to loosen mucus and clear the respiratory tract, easing congestion and promoting sinus drainage. Inhalation of Eucalyptus oil can also provide a cooling sensation and relieve headaches often associated with sinusitis.

Peppermint essential oil is another popular choice for sinusitis relief. It has a cooling and invigorating effect and is known for its ability to alleviate congestion and reduce headaches. Peppermint oil contains menthol, which helps to open up the airways and improve breathing. It can be applied topically to the chest or temples, or inhaled through steam inhalation.

Tea Tree essential oil is valued for its antibacterial and antifungal properties. It can help fight off microbial infections that contribute to sinusitis and reduce inflammation in the nasal passages. Tea Tree oil can be diffused in the air or applied topically with a carrier oil to help alleviate symptoms and support the body's natural healing processes.

Lavender essential oil, known for its calming and relaxing properties, can also be beneficial for sinusitis. While it may not directly address congestion, it can help reduce stress and promote better sleep, which can support overall wellness and aid in recovery from sinusitis. Lavender oil can be diffused in the bedroom or added to a warm bath for its soothing effects.

When using aromatherapy for sinusitis, it's important to consider safety precautions and proper usage. Essential oils are highly concentrated and should be used with caution. It's advisable to dilute essential oils with a carrier oil, such as coconut or almond oil, before applying them to the skin to prevent irritation or sensitization. Additionally, some essential oils may interact with certain medications, so it's essential to consult a healthcare professional if you have any underlying health conditions or are taking medications.

Aromatherapy can be enjoyed through various methods, including diffusers, inhalation, and topical application. Diffusers disperse essential oils into the air, allowing you to inhale the aromatic molecules. Steam inhalation, where a few drops of essential oil are added to hot water, can provide targeted relief for sinusitis symptoms. Topical application involves diluting essential oils with a carrier oil and applying the mixture to the skin, usually on the chest.

Chapter Twenty-Three

Sinusitis and the Weather

The Impact of Weather on Sinusitis: Exploring the Connection

Sinusitis, a condition characterized by inflammation of the sinus cavities, can be a frustrating and uncomfortable experience. While it is primarily caused by factors such as allergies, infections, or anatomical issues, many individuals also report that weather changes can trigger or worsen their sinusitis symptoms. Below we will explore the relationship between sinusitis and the weather, examining the potential impact of various weather conditions on sinus health and discussing strategies for managing symptoms.

Weather conditions, such as changes in temperature, humidity, and barometric pressure, have long been associated with the onset or exacerbation of sinusitis symptoms. While the exact mechanisms underlying this relationship are not fully understood, several theories have been proposed to explain why weather changes can affect sinus health.

One of the main factors that impact sinusitis symptoms is humidity. Dry air can cause the nasal passages to become dry and irritated, leading to congestion, discomfort, and an increased risk of infection. On the other hand, high humidity can contribute to the growth of mold, dust mites, and other allergens that can trigger sinusitis symptoms in individuals who are sensitive to them. Therefore, both extremely dry and excessively humid weather conditions can be problematic for those with sinusitis.

Temperature fluctuations also play a role in sinus health. Cold temperatures can cause blood vessels in the nasal passages to constrict, leading to reduced blood flow and potentially worsening congestion. In contrast, warmer temperatures can cause blood vessels to dilate, which may increase mucus production and contribute to nasal congestion. Additionally, sudden changes in temperature, such as going from a warm environment to a cold one, can trigger sinusitis symptoms in some individuals.

Barometric pressure, the atmospheric pressure exerted on the body, is another weather, related factor that can impact sinusitis symptoms. Changes in barometric pressure, often associated with weather fronts, can cause the air pressure within the sinuses to become imbalanced, leading to pain and discomfort. Some individuals report increased sinus pain and pressure before or during a weather change, such as the arrival of a storm or a rapid shift in atmospheric pressure.

Mañaging sinusitis symptoms in relation to weather changes requires a proactive approach. Here are some strategies that can help individuals cope with the impact of weather on sinus health:

Stay hydrated: Drinking plenty of fluids helps to keep the nasal passages moist and prevent excessive dryness. It is especially important to drink water when in dry or heated environments.

Use nasal saline rinses: Nasal saline rinses help to moisturize the nasal passages and flush out irritants and allergens. They can be particularly beneficial during dry or dusty weather conditions.

Maintain a comfortable indoor environment: Using a humidifier or vaporizer can add moisture to the air, preventing dryness in the nasal passages. Additionally, using air purifiers can help filter out allergens and pollutants that may exacerbate sinusitis symptoms.

Dress appropriately for the weather: Protecting the nasal area with a scarf or a mask can help reduce the impact of cold air on the nasal passages. Dressing in layers can also help manage temperature fluctuations.

Manage allergies: If you have allergies that contribute to your sinusitis symptoms, it is important to take steps to minimize exposure to allergens. This may include regularly cleaning your living space, using allergen, proof covers for bedding, and avoiding outdoor activities during times when allergen levels are high.

Seek medical advice: If your sinusitis symptoms are significantly impacted by weather changes, it may be beneficial to consult with a healthcare professional. They can provide personalized recommendations and may suggest additional treatments or interventions to manage your symptoms.

Weather Changes and Sinus Pressure

The Connection between Weather Changes and Sinus Pressure: Exploring the Impact

Sinus pressure, a common symptom of sinusitis, can cause discomfort and affect our daily lives. Many individuals with sinusitis notice that their symptoms, particularly sinus pressure, worsen during certain weather conditions or weather changes. Below we will delve into the relationship between weather changes and sinus pressure, examining the potential factors involved and discussing strategies to manage this phenomenon effectively.

Weather changes, including shifts in temperature, humidity, and barometric pressure, have been identified as potential triggers for sinus pressure. While the exact mechanisms are not fully understood, several theories have been proposed to explain this connection.

Temperature fluctuations can play a role in sinus pressure. Cold weather can cause the blood vessels in the nasal passages to constrict, leading to decreased blood flow and increased pressure. This constriction can result in congestion and a feeling of heaviness in the sinuses. On the other hand, warm weather can cause the blood vessels to dilate, leading to increased blood flow and potential swelling of the sinus tissues, contributing to sinus pressure.

Humidity levels also impact sinus pressure. Dry air can dry out the nasal passages, leading to irritation and inflammation. This can cause the nasal tissues to swell, leading to increased pressure and discomfort. In contrast, high humidity can contribute to an environment where mold, dust mites, and other allergens thrive. For individuals sensitive to these allergens, exposure can trigger inflammation and worsen sinus pressure.

Barometric pressure, the atmospheric pressure exerted on the body, is another significant factor in sinus pressure during weather changes. When a weather front approaches or changes, such as before a storm, there may be a rapid shift in barometric pressure. This can disrupt the pressure balance within the sinuses, leading to a feeling of fullness, pain, and pressure.

Managing sinus pressure during weather changes requires proactive measures. Here are some strategies that can help individuals alleviate and prevent sinus pressure:

Stay hydrated: Drinking plenty of fluids helps to keep the nasal passages moist and prevents dryness. Adequate hydration can help reduce nasal irritation and alleviate sinus pressure.

Use nasal saline rinses: Nasal saline rinses provide moisture to the nasal passages and help flush out irritants and allergens. Regular use can help alleviate congestion and reduce sinus pressure.

Apply warm compresses: Placing warm compresses on the face can help soothe the nasal passages and promote sinus drainage. This can provide relief from sinus pressure and congestion.

Use over, the, counter nasal decongestants: Nasal decongestant sprays or nasal drops can provide temporary relief from sinus pressure by constricting the blood vessels in the nasal passages. However, prolonged use should be avoided, as it can lead to rebound congestion.

Practice sinus irrigation: Neti pots or sinus irrigation systems can be used to rinse the nasal passages with a saline solution. This helps to clear mucus, reduce inflammation, and alleviate sinus pressure.

Manage allergies: If allergies contribute to sinus pressure, it is important to identify and manage allergens effectively. This may involve avoiding triggers, using allergy medications, or seeking allergen immunotherapy under the guidance of a healthcare professional.

Monitor weather forecasts: Pay attention to weather forecasts and be prepared for weather changes that may trigger sinus pressure. Taking preventive measures ahead of time, such as using nasal sprays or applying warm compresses, can help reduce the impact of weather, related sinus pressure.

Seek medical advice: If sinus pressure becomes severe or persistent, it is advisable to consult a healthcare professional. They can assess your condition, provide appropriate treatment options, and offer further guidance on managing sinus pressure during weather changes.

Coping with Seasonal Sinusitis

Coping with Seasonal Sinusitis: Strategies for Managing Symptoms

Sinusitis, an inflammation of the sinuses, can be particularly challenging during certain seasons. Seasonal changes, such as spring and fall, can trigger sinusitis symptoms due to increased pollen levels, temperature fluctuations, and other environmental factors. Below we will explore effective strategies for coping with seasonal sinusitis and managing its symptoms to maintain a good quality of life.

Understand your triggers: Identifying the specific triggers that worsen your sinusitis symptoms during certain seasons is crucial. For many individuals, pollen from trees, grasses, and weeds is a common allergen that can exacerbate sinusitis. By knowing your triggers, you can take proactive steps to minimize exposure and manage symptoms effectively.

Monitor pollen counts: Keep track of local pollen counts and plan your activities accordingly. On days when pollen levels are high, consider staying indoors or limiting your time outdoors, particularly during peak pollen hours. You can find local pollen forecasts online or through various weather apps.

Create an allergen, free home: Make your home a safe haven from allergens by implementing certain measures. Keep windows closed during high pollen seasons and use air purifiers with HEPA filters to reduce airborne allergens. Regularly vacuum and dust your home to minimize dust mites and other allergens that can worsen sinusitis symptoms.

Use nasal saline rinses: Nasal saline rinses, such as neti pots or saline nasal sprays, help flush out allergens, mucus, and irritants from the nasal passages. Regular use can alleviate congestion, reduce inflammation, and promote sinus drainage, providing relief from seasonal sinusitis symptoms.

Take allergy medications: Over, the, counter or prescription allergy medications can help manage seasonal allergies and minimize sinusitis symptoms. Antihistamines, nasal corticosteroids, and decongestants are commonly used to relieve congestion, reduce inflammation, and alleviate discomfort.

Practice good hygiene: Maintaining good hygiene can help prevent the spread of allergens and irritants. Wash your hands frequently, especially after being outdoors, to remove pollen and other allergens from your skin. Avoid touching your face, particularly your eyes and nose, to minimize contact with allergens.

Use protective gear: When participating in outdoor activities during high pollen seasons, consider wearing a hat, sunglasses, and a pollen mask or respirator. These can provide an additional barrier against allergens and reduce the risk of triggering sinusitis symptoms.

Manage indoor humidity: Keep indoor humidity levels between 30% and 50% to prevent the growth of mold and dust mites, which can worsen sinusitis symptoms. Use a dehumidifier or air conditioner, particularly in damp areas like the basement, to control humidity levels.

Support your immune system: Maintaining a healthy immune system can help reduce the frequency and severity of sinusitis symptoms. Eat a balanced diet rich in fruits, vegetables, whole grains, and lean proteins. Stay physically active, get enough sleep, and manage stress effectively to support your immune system.

Seek medical advice: If your sinusitis symptoms persist or worsen despite self, care measures, it is important to seek medical advice. A healthcare professional can evaluate your condition, provide a proper diagnosis, and recommend appropriate treatment options to manage seasonal sinusitis effectively.

Consider immunotherapy: For individuals with severe seasonal allergies and recurrent sinusitis, allergen immunotherapy may be an option. This treatment involves exposing the body to small amounts of allergens to build tolerance over time. It can help reduce sensitivity to allergens and minimize sinusitis symptoms.

Sinusitis in Extreme Climates

Sinusitis in Extreme Climates: Understanding and Managing Symptoms

Sinusitis, an inflammation of the sinuses, can affect individuals living in various climates, including those with extreme weather conditions. Whether it's the dry and arid deserts or the cold and frigid regions, extreme climates can pose unique challenges for sinus health. Below we will explore the impact of extreme climates on sinusitis and discuss effective strategies for managing symptoms in such environments.

Dry and Arid Climates:

In dry and arid climates, low humidity levels can exacerbate sinusitis symptoms. The lack of moisture in the air can cause the nasal passages to become dry and irritated, leading to congestion, discomfort, and increased susceptibility to infections. Here are some tips for managing sinusitis in dry climates:

a. Use a humidifier: Installing a humidifier in your home can help add moisture to the air and prevent dryness of the nasal passages. This can alleviate congestion and reduce the risk of sinusitis flare, ups.

b. Stay hydrated: Drink plenty of fluids to stay hydrated and keep the nasal passages moist. Water, herbal teas, and clear broths can help maintain adequate hydration levels.

c. Nasal saline rinses: Regularly irrigating the nasal passages with saline solution can help moisturize and cleanse the nasal cavities. This can reduce congestion and alleviate sinusitis symptoms.

d. Avoid irritants: In dry climates, irritants such as dust, smoke, and strong chemicals can worsen sinusitis symptoms. Minimize exposure to these irritants by using air purifiers and wearing a mask when necessary.

Cold and Frigid Climates:

Cold and frigid climates present their own challenges for individuals with sinusitis. The cold weather and low temperatures can lead to vasoconstriction of the blood vessels in the nasal passages, reducing blood flow and causing nasal congestion. Additionally, spending time indoors in heated environments can result in dry air, further aggravating sinusitis symptoms. Here are some strategies for managing sinusitis in cold climates:

a. Keep warm: Protect your nose and face from cold temperatures by wearing a scarf or a mask that covers your nose and mouth. This can help warm the air before it reaches your nasal passages, reducing the risk of congestion.

b. Use a humidifier: In heated indoor environments, use a humidifier to add moisture to the air and prevent dryness of the nasal passages. This can alleviate congestion and reduce discomfort.

c. Stay hydrated: Drink ample fluids to stay hydrated, even if you don't feel as thirsty in colder climates. Hydration is crucial for maintaining the moisture levels in your nasal passages.

d. Nasal saline rinses: Regularly flushing your nasal passages with saline solution can help remove mucus, allergens, and irritants, keeping your sinuses clear and reducing congestion.

High Altitude Climates:

High altitude climates, such as mountainous regions, pose unique challenges for individuals with sinusitis. At higher elevations, the air pressure decreases, which can affect the sinuses and cause discomfort. Additionally, changes in altitude during travel can lead to barotrauma, resulting in pain and pressure in the sinuses. Here are some tips for managing sinusitis in high altitude climates:

a. Stay hydrated: Drinking plenty of fluids helps maintain hydration and keeps the nasal passages moist. This can alleviate symptoms associated with dryness and congestion.

b. Take frequent breaks during travel: If you're traveling to higher altitudes, allow yourself time to acclimate. Gradually ascend to higher elevations, taking breaks as needed to adjust to the changes in pressure.

Chapter Twenty-Four

Sinusitis and Travel

Sinusitis and Travel: Tips for a Smooth Journey

Sinusitis, an inflammation of the sinuses, can cause discomfort and inconvenience, especially when traveling. Whether you're taking a short road trip or embarking on a long, haul flight, the changes in pressure, air quality, and environmental factors can affect your sinus health. Below we will explore the impact of travel on sinusitis and provide useful tips for managing symptoms and ensuring a smooth journey.

Air Travel and Sinusitis:

Air travel can present unique challenges for individuals with sinusitis due to the changes in air pressure during takeoff, landing, and altitude variations. Here are some tips to help manage sinusitis symptoms while flying:

a. Nasal saline sprays: Use saline nasal sprays before and during the flight to keep your nasal passages moisturized. This can help alleviate congestion and prevent dryness.

b. Stay hydrated: Drink plenty of water before and during the flight to stay hydrated. Avoid excessive caffeine and alcohol, as they can contribute to dehydration.

c. Use decongestants cautiously: If necessary, consult your healthcare provider before using decongestant medications. They can help reduce congestion, but they should be used with caution and according to instructions.

d. Practice swallowing and yawning: Swallowing or yawning can help equalize the pressure in your ears and sinuses. Chew gum or suck on a candy to encourage swallowing during takeoff and landing.

e. Consider using earplugs: Special earplugs designed for air travel can help regulate air pressure changes and minimize discomfort. Consult with your healthcare provider or pharmacist for recommendations.

Road Trips and Sinusitis:

Road trips can be enjoyable, but long hours spent in a vehicle can exacerbate sinusitis symptoms. Here are some tips for managing sinusitis during road trips:

a. Maintain air circulation: Keep the car well, ventilated to ensure fresh air circulation. Use air conditioning or open the windows periodically to prevent stuffiness.

b. Use a humidifier: If possible, use a portable humidifier in the car to add moisture to the air. This can help prevent dryness and reduce nasal congestion.

c. Take breaks: Regularly stop the car and stretch your legs. Use these breaks as an opportunity to walk around and breathe in fresh air.

d. Stay hydrated: Drink plenty of water during the road trip to stay hydrated. This helps maintain the moisture levels in your nasal passages and reduce discomfort.

Traveling to Different Climates:

Traveling to different climates can have an impact on sinusitis symptoms. Changes in temperature, humidity, and allergen exposure can trigger flare, ups. Here are some tips to manage sinusitis while traveling to different climates:

a. Research the climate: Before your trip, research the weather conditions and allergen levels at your destination. This will help you prepare and take necessary precautions.

b. Pack appropriate medications: Ensure you have an adequate supply of your prescribed medications, including nasal sprays, antihistamines, or decongestants. If you use a humidifier or nasal irrigations, consider packing portable versions.

c. Protect yourself from allergens: If you're traveling to an area with known allergens, such as pollen or dust mites, take steps to minimize exposure. Close windows in hotel rooms, use air purifiers if available, and avoid outdoor activities during peak allergen times.

d. Manage your stress levels: Stress can contribute to sinusitis symptoms. Engage in relaxation techniques such as deep breathing exercises, meditation, or listening to calming music to reduce stress while traveling.

Managing Sinusitis While Traveling

Managing Sinusitis While Traveling: Tips for a Smooth Journey

Traveling can be an exciting adventure, but for individuals with sinusitis, it can also bring challenges. Sinusitis, an inflammation of the sinuses, can cause discomfort and disrupt your travel plans. However, with proper management and preparation, you can minimize symptoms and ensure a smooth journey. Below we will explore practical tips for managing sinusitis while traveling, allowing you to make the most of your travel experience.

Plan Ahead:

Before embarking on your trip, it's important to plan ahead and take certain precautions:

a. Consult with your healthcare provider: If you have chronic sinusitis or frequent sinus infections, consult with your healthcare provider before traveling. They can provide guidance, prescribe medications if necessary, and offer personalized advice based on your specific condition.

b. Pack essential medications: Ensure you have an adequate supply of your prescribed medications for the duration of your trip. This may include nasal sprays, decongestants, antihistamines, or antibiotics. Remember to pack them in your carry, on bag for easy access during the journey.

c. Research your destination: Research the climate and environmental conditions at your destination. Knowing the weather patterns, allergen levels, and air quality can help you prepare and take necessary precautions.

Manage Sinus Symptoms:

To manage sinusitis symptoms while traveling, consider the following tips:

a. Maintain nasal hygiene: Regularly rinse your nasal passages with saline solution or use a nasal irrigator. This helps remove irritants, moisturizes the sinuses, and reduces congestion.

b. Stay hydrated: Drink plenty of water during your journey to keep your nasal passages moisturized. Avoid excessive caffeine and alcohol, as they can contribute to dehydration.

c. Use nasal sprays: Over, the, counter saline nasal sprays can provide temporary relief by moisturizing the nasal passages and reducing congestion. Use them as directed or as recommended by your healthcare provider.

d. Practice sinus pressure equalization: During takeoff and landing on flights or when changing altitudes, practice techniques such as swallowing, yawning, or gently blowing through your nose while pinching it closed. This helps equalize pressure and prevent discomfort.

Air Travel Considerations:

Air travel can pose specific challenges for individuals with sinusitis. Here are some tips to make your air travel more comfortable:

a. Choose the right seat: Opt for a seat that allows you to elevate your head slightly, such as an aisle or bulkhead seat. This can help reduce congestion and prevent sinus pressure buildup.

b. Use a nasal decongestant: If approved by your healthcare provider, consider using a nasal decongestant spray before boarding the plane. This can help alleviate congestion and improve airflow.

c. Keep nasal passages moist: Use a saline nasal spray or apply a thin layer of petroleum jelly inside your nostrils to help retain moisture during the flight. This can prevent dryness and irritation.

d. Stay active during the flight: Walk around the cabin, stretch your legs, and perform gentle neck and shoulder exercises to promote blood circulation and prevent stiffness.

Minimize Allergen Exposure:

Allergens can exacerbate sinusitis symptoms, so it's important to minimize exposure while traveling:

a. Research local allergens: If you're traveling to a region known for specific allergens, such as pollen or mold, research the local allergen season and take appropriate precautions. This may include avoiding outdoor activities during peak allergen times or wearing a mask in high, pollen areas.

b. Use allergen, proof bedding: If you're staying in accommodations where allergens may be present, such as dust mites or pet dander, consider using allergen, proof bedding covers to reduce exposure.

Travel Tips for Sinusitis Sufferers

Travel Tips for Sinusitis Sufferers: Enjoying Your Journey with Ease

Traveling can be an exciting and fulfilling experience, but for individuals with sinusitis, it can also present challenges. Sinusitis, characterized by inflammation of the sinuses, can cause discomfort and affect your travel plans. However, with proper preparation and some practical tips, you can manage your sinusitis symptoms and enjoy a smooth journey. Below we will explore helpful travel tips for sinusitis sufferers, ensuring that your travel experience is as pleasant as possible.

Consult with Your Healthcare Provider:

Before embarking on your trip, it's essential to consult with your healthcare provider, especially if you have chronic sinusitis or a history of frequent sinus infections. They can provide personalized advice and recommendations based on your specific condition. Additionally, they can review your medications, prescribe any necessary treatments or antibiotics, and ensure you are well, prepared for your journey.

Plan and Pack Strategically:

Proper planning and packing are crucial for managing sinusitis while traveling. Consider the following tips:

a. Research your destination: Before your trip, research the climate and environmental conditions at your destination. This information can help you anticipate potential triggers and plan accordingly.

b. Pack essential medications: Make sure to pack an adequate supply of your prescribed medications, including nasal sprays, decongestants, and antihistamines. Keep them easily accessible in your carry, on bag in case you need them during the journey.

c. Carry a doctor's letter: If you are carrying medications or medical devices such as nasal sprays, it can be helpful to have a doctor's letter outlining your condition and the necessity of these items. This can assist in navigating security checkpoints without any issues.

d. Use travel, friendly packaging: To save space and make packing easier, transfer your medications and nasal sprays into travel, sized containers. Additionally, consider using a pill organizer to keep your medications organized and easily accessible throughout your trip.

Manage Sinusitis Symptoms:

Effectively managing your sinusitis symptoms is essential to ensure a comfortable journey. Here are some tips:

a. Keep nasal passages moisturized: Dry nasal passages can worsen sinusitis symptoms. Use saline nasal sprays or saline rinses to moisturize and cleanse your nasal passages regularly. This helps reduce congestion and alleviate discomfort.

b. Stay hydrated: Drink plenty of water throughout your journey to keep your body hydrated. This helps thin the mucus in your sinuses and promotes better drainage.

c. Avoid triggers: Identify and avoid triggers that can worsen your sinusitis symptoms. These may include allergens, pollutants, or certain foods. If you're traveling to an area with high allergen levels, consider wearing a mask or limiting your outdoor activities during peak pollen times.

d. Practice good hygiene: Wash your hands frequently to reduce the risk of infections. Avoid touching your face, especially your nose and eyes, to prevent the spread of bacteria or viruses.

Choose Travel Methods Wisely:

The mode of transportation you choose can impact your sinusitis symptoms. Consider the following tips:

a. Air travel considerations: If you are traveling by air, changes in cabin pressure during takeoff and landing can affect your sinuses. To minimize discomfort, swallow, yawn, or chew gum to equalize the pressure in your ears and sinuses. Additionally, using a nasal decongestant spray before boarding can help reduce congestion.

b. Road trip preparations: If you're embarking on a road trip, ensure your vehicle is clean and free from dust and allergens. Keep the windows closed and use the air conditioning system with a clean air filter to maintain a controlled environment inside the car.

Coping with Altitude Changes

Coping with Altitude Changes: Managing Sinusitis in High, Altitude Environments

Altitude changes can have a significant impact on our bodies, especially for individuals with sinusitis. The change in atmospheric pressure and oxygen levels can exacerbate sinus symptoms and lead to discomfort. However, with proper understanding and some practical strategies, it is possible to cope with altitude changes and manage sinusitis effectively. Below we will explore tips and techniques for managing sinusitis in high, altitude environments, ensuring a more comfortable experience for individuals with this condition.

Understanding Altitude Changes:

Before delving into coping strategies, it's important to understand how altitude changes affect our sinuses. As we ascend to higher altitudes, the atmospheric pressure decreases. This change can cause the air inside our sinuses to expand, resulting in increased pressure and potential pain. Additionally, the lower oxygen levels at higher altitudes can lead to decreased blood flow and oxygen supply to the sinuses, further aggravating symptoms.

Gradual Acclimatization:

One of the key strategies for coping with altitude changes is gradual acclimatization. If possible, give your body time to adjust to the new altitude gradually. This approach allows your sinuses to adapt and minimizes the discomfort associated with sudden changes in pressure. Here are some tips for gradual acclimatization:

a. Ascend slowly: When traveling to higher altitudes, try to ascend gradually instead of making rapid changes in elevation. This can be particularly important if you are traveling to a significantly higher altitude. Gradually increasing your altitude over a few days allows your body to adjust and adapt to the changes.

b. Take rest breaks: If you are engaging in activities such as hiking or climbing at high altitudes, take regular rest breaks to give your body time to adjust. Use this time to hydrate, relax, and allow your sinuses to acclimate to the new environment.

c. Monitor your symptoms: Pay attention to any changes in your sinus symptoms during the acclimatization process. If you notice increased discomfort or severe symptoms, consider descending to a lower altitude or seeking medical attention.

Stay Hydrated:

Proper hydration is crucial for managing sinusitis in high, altitude environments. The dry air at higher altitudes can cause dehydration and exacerbate sinus symptoms. Here are some hydration tips:

a. Drink plenty of water: Increase your fluid intake to stay hydrated. Carry a reusable water bottle with you and sip water frequently throughout the day.

b. Avoid alcohol and caffeine: Limit your consumption of alcohol and caffeine, as they can contribute to dehydration. Instead, opt for water, herbal tea, or electrolyte, rich beverages.

c. Use saline nasal sprays: Regularly using saline nasal sprays helps keep your nasal passages moisturized and prevents dryness. This can alleviate sinus congestion and discomfort.

Nasal Irrigation:

Nasal irrigation is an effective technique for managing sinusitis symptoms in high, altitude environments. It involves flushing out the sinuses with a saline solution to remove mucus, allergens, and irritants. This can help relieve congestion and promote sinus health. Here's how to perform nasal irrigation:

a. Prepare a saline solution: Mix a teaspoon of non, iodized salt with a cup of warm distilled or boiled water. Ensure the solution is well, mixed and free from any impurities.

b. Use a neti pot or nasal irrigation bottle: Fill the neti pot or irrigation bottle with the saline solution. Tilt your head to the side over a sink and pour the solution into one nostril while breathing through your mouth.

Allow the solution to flow through your nasal passages and out the other nostril.

Chapter Twenty-Five

Pregnancy and Sinusitis

Pregnancy and Sinusitis: Understanding the Challenges and Management

Pregnancy is a remarkable journey filled with various physical changes and challenges. One common issue that some pregnant women may face is sinusitis, which refers to the inflammation of the sinus cavities. Sinusitis during pregnancy can be a discomforting experience, but with proper understanding and management, it can be effectively addressed. Below we will explore the relationship between pregnancy and sinusitis, the challenges it poses, and the appropriate strategies for managing sinusitis during this special time.

Understanding Sinusitis During Pregnancy:

Sinusitis can occur during pregnancy due to hormonal changes, increased blood volume, and nasal congestion. The hormonal changes, particularly the rise in estrogen levels, can cause the blood vessels in the nasal passages to swell, leading to congestion and inflammation. The increased blood volume can also contribute to nasal congestion, making pregnant women more susceptible to sinusitis.

Common Symptoms and Challenges:

The symptoms of sinusitis during pregnancy are similar to those experienced by non, pregnant individuals and may include:

a. Nasal congestion: Pregnant women may experience difficulty breathing through the nose due to nasal congestion. This can lead to a feeling of stuffiness and discomfort.

b. Facial pain and pressure: Sinusitis can cause pain and pressure in the face, particularly around the forehead, cheeks, and eyes.

c. Headache: Sinus headaches may occur as a result of sinus inflammation and congestion.

d. Postnasal drip: Excess mucus production can lead to postnasal drip, causing a sensation of mucus dripping down the throat.

e. Cough: Sinus drainage can trigger a persistent cough.

Challenges in managing sinusitis during pregnancy include the limited treatment options available due to safety concerns for the developing fetus. Many over, the, counter medications and even some prescription medications may not be recommended during pregnancy, requiring alternative approaches for relief.

Consultation with Healthcare Provider:

If you suspect you have sinusitis during pregnancy, it is important to consult with your healthcare provider. They can evaluate your symptoms, provide a proper diagnosis, and recommend suitable treatment options. It is crucial to inform your healthcare provider about your pregnancy to ensure that any treatment recommendations are safe for both you and your baby.

Natural Remedies for Symptom Relief:

Since medication options may be limited during pregnancy, natural remedies can provide relief from sinusitis symptoms. Here are some safe and effective natural remedies for managing sinusitis:

a. Nasal saline irrigation: Using a saline solution to rinse the nasal passages can help relieve congestion and remove irritants. Use a neti pot or a saline nasal spray to perform nasal irrigation.

b. Steam inhalation: Inhaling steam from a bowl of hot water or using a humidifier can help moisturize the nasal passages and alleviate congestion.

c. Warm compress: Applying a warm compress to the face can help relieve facial pain and pressure associated with sinusitis.

d. Rest and hydration: Getting plenty of rest and staying hydrated can support your body's natural healing process and reduce symptoms.

Lifestyle Modifications:

In addition to natural remedies, certain lifestyle modifications can contribute to managing sinusitis during pregnancy:

a. Maintain proper hydration: Drinking an adequate amount of water can help thin mucus and alleviate congestion.

b. Use a humidifier: Adding moisture to the air with a humidifier can reduce nasal dryness and ease congestion.

c. Avoid allergens and irritants: Identify and avoid any triggers that worsen your sinus symptoms, such as smoke, strong odors, and allergens like dust or pet dander.

d. Elevate your head during sleep: Using an extra pillow or sleeping with an elevated head position can promote sinus drainage and alleviate congestion.

Sinusitis During Pregnancy

Sinusitis During Pregnancy: Understanding the Challenges and Management

Pregnancy is a remarkable journey filled with joy and anticipation. However, along with the beautiful changes that occur in a woman's body, there may be some challenges as well. One common issue that some pregnant women may face is sinusitis, which refers to the inflammation of the sinus cavities. Sinusitis during pregnancy can be discomforting, but with proper understanding and management, it can be effectively addressed. Below we will explore the relationship between pregnancy and sinusitis, the challenges it poses, and the appropriate strategies for managing sinusitis during this special time.

Understanding Sinusitis During Pregnancy:

Sinusitis is a condition characterized by the inflammation of the sinus cavities, which are the air, filled spaces within the facial bones surrounding the nose. During pregnancy, hormonal changes, increased blood volume, and nasal congestion can contribute to the development of sinusitis. The rise in hormone levels, particularly estrogen, can cause the blood vessels in the nasal passages to swell, leading to congestion and inflammation. The increased blood volume can also contribute to nasal congestion, making pregnant women more susceptible to sinusitis.

Common Symptoms and Challenges:

The symptoms of sinusitis during pregnancy are similar to those experienced by non, pregnant individuals and may include:

a. Nasal congestion: Pregnant women may experience difficulty breathing through the nose due to nasal congestion. This can lead to a feeling of stuffiness and discomfort.

b. Facial pain and pressure: Sinusitis can cause pain and pressure in the face, particularly around the forehead, cheeks, and eyes.

c. Headache: Sinus headaches may occur as a result of sinus inflammation and congestion.

d. Postnasal drip: Excess mucus production can lead to postnasal drip, causing a sensation of mucus dripping down the throat.

e. Cough: Sinus drainage can trigger a persistent cough.

Challenges in managing sinusitis during pregnancy include the limited treatment options available due to safety concerns for the developing fetus. Many over, the, counter medications and even some prescription medications may not be recommended during pregnancy, requiring alternative approaches for relief.

Consultation with Healthcare Provider:

If you suspect you have sinusitis during pregnancy, it is important to consult with your healthcare provider. They can evaluate your symptoms, provide a proper diagnosis, and recommend suitable treatment options. It is crucial to inform your healthcare provider about your pregnancy to ensure that any treatment recommendations are safe for both you and your baby.

Natural Remedies for Symptom Relief:

Since medication options may be limited during pregnancy, natural remedies can provide relief from sinusitis symptoms. Here are some safe and effective natural remedies for managing sinusitis:

a. Nasal saline irrigation: Using a saline solution to rinse the nasal passages can help relieve congestion and remove irritants. Use a neti pot or a saline nasal spray to perform nasal irrigation.

b. Steam inhalation: Inhaling steam from a bowl of hot water or using a humidifier can help moisturize the nasal passages and alleviate congestion.

c. Warm compress: Applying a warm compress to the face can help relieve facial pain and pressure associated with sinusitis.

d. Rest and hydration: Getting plenty of rest and staying hydrated can support your body's natural healing process and reduce symptoms.

Lifestyle Modifications:

In addition to natural remedies, certain lifestyle modifications can contribute to managing sinusitis during pregnancy:

a. Maintain proper hydration: Drinking an adequate amount of water can help thin mucus and alleviate congestion.

b. Use a humidifier: Adding moisture to the air with a humidifier can reduce nasal dryness and ease congestion.

c. Avoid allergens and irritants: Identify and avoid any triggers that worsen your sinus symptoms, such as smoke.

Safe Treatments for Pregnant Women

Sinusitis is a common condition that can occur during pregnancy, causing discomfort and potential complications. When it comes to treating sinusitis in pregnant women, safety is a top priority. It is essential to choose treatments that are effective and pose minimal risk to both the mother and the developing baby. Below we will explore safe treatment options for pregnant women with sinusitis, focusing on those that have been deemed safe by healthcare professionals.

Consultation with a Healthcare Provider:

The first step in managing sinusitis during pregnancy is to consult with a healthcare provider. They will evaluate your symptoms and medical history to provide appropriate guidance and treatment recommendations. This is particularly important during pregnancy, as some medications and interventions may carry potential risks to the developing baby. Your healthcare provider will consider your individual circumstances to ensure the safety and efficacy of any treatment options.

Nasal Saline Irrigation:

Nasal saline irrigation is a safe and effective method to alleviate symptoms of sinusitis during pregnancy. It involves rinsing the nasal passages with a saline solution to help clear mucus, reduce congestion, and promote sinus drainage. This technique is generally well, tolerated and can be performed using a neti pot or a saline nasal spray. Nasal saline irrigation provides relief without the use of medications, making it a preferred option for pregnant women.

Steam Inhalation:

Steam inhalation is another safe and natural remedy for sinusitis during pregnancy. Inhaling steam helps moisturize the nasal passages, reduce inflammation, and alleviate congestion. To practice steam inhalation, simply fill a bowl with hot water and place your face above the bowl, covering your head with a towel to trap the steam. Breathe deeply for several minutes to experience the soothing effects. Alternatively, using a humidifier in your living space can provide consistent moisture and help relieve sinusitis symptoms.

Warm Compresses:

Applying warm compresses to the affected areas of the face can provide temporary relief from facial pain and pressure associated with sinusitis.

The warmth helps to reduce inflammation and promote sinus drainage. You can make a warm compress by soaking a clean towel in warm water and placing it on your face, focusing on the sinus areas. Repeat this process several times a day to ease discomfort.

Rest and Hydration:

Getting ample rest and staying hydrated are essential components of managing sinusitis during pregnancy. Rest allows your body to heal and recover, while hydration helps to thin mucus and prevent congestion. Make sure to drink plenty of water throughout the day to maintain proper hydration levels. Additionally, incorporating healthy fluids such as herbal teas and warm broths can also provide relief.

Natural Remedies:

Certain natural remedies can be safely used to alleviate sinusitis symptoms in pregnant women. These include:

a. Steam inhalation with essential oils: Adding a few drops of essential oils such as eucalyptus or peppermint to the hot water used for steam inhalation can enhance the benefits. However, it is crucial to consult with a healthcare provider or a certified aromatherapist to ensure the safe use of essential oils during pregnancy.

b. Warm saline gargles: Gargling with warm saline water can help soothe a sore throat and reduce postnasal drip associated with sinusitis. Mix half a teaspoon of salt in a cup of warm water and gargle for 30 seconds, then spit it out. Repeat several times a day as needed.

c. Elevating the head while sleeping: Using extra pillows or a wedge pillow to elevate the head while sleeping can promote better sinus drainage and alleviate congestion during the night.

Avoidance of Potential Triggers:

Pregnant women with sinusitis should be mindful of potential triggers that can worsen symptoms.

Prevention Tips for Expecting Mothers

Sinusitis, an inflammation of the sinuses, can be particularly uncomfortable for expecting mothers. Pregnancy alters the immune system and hormonal balance, making pregnant women more susceptible to sinusitis. However, there are preventive measures that can help minimize the risk of developing sinusitis during pregnancy. Below we will explore effective prevention tips for expecting mothers to maintain sinus health and reduce the likelihood of sinusitis.

Maintain Good Hygiene:

Practicing good hygiene is crucial in preventing sinusitis. Wash your hands frequently with soap and water to minimize the spread of germs that can cause sinus infections. Avoid touching your face, especially your nose and eyes, as it can introduce bacteria and viruses into the sinuses.

Stay Hydrated:

Proper hydration is essential for overall health, including sinus health. Drinking an adequate amount of water throughout the day helps to keep nasal passages moist and thin mucus, reducing the risk of sinusitis. Aim for at least eight glasses of water per day, and consider incorporating hydrating fluids such as herbal teas and fresh juices into your daily routine.

Maintain a Clean Living Environment:

Creating a clean and healthy living environment can significantly reduce the risk of sinusitis. Regularly clean and dust your home to minimize exposure to allergens and irritants that can trigger sinus inflammation. Vacuum carpets and upholstery, change air filters, and keep indoor humidity levels in check to prevent mold growth.

Manage Allergies:

Allergies can exacerbate sinusitis symptoms, so it's important to manage them effectively during pregnancy. Identify your allergens and take necessary steps to avoid exposure to them. Keep windows closed during high pollen seasons, use allergen, proof bedding covers, and consider using a HEPA filter in your home to reduce airborne allergens.

Avoid Irritants:

Certain irritants, such as cigarette smoke and strong chemical odors, can irritate the nasal passages and trigger sinusitis. As an expecting mother, it is essential to stay away from such irritants to maintain sinus health. Avoid secondhand smoke and choose natural, fragrance, free products for cleaning and personal care.

Practice Nasal Irrigation:

Nasal irrigation with saline solution can help keep nasal passages clean and clear, reducing the risk of sinusitis. Use a neti pot or a saline nasal spray to flush out irritants, allergens, and excess mucus from the nasal passages. However, it's crucial to follow proper hygiene and use sterile saline solution to prevent any contamination.

Use a Humidifier:

Maintaining proper humidity levels in your home can help keep nasal passages moist and prevent sinus congestion. Consider using a humidifier, especially during dry winter months or in environments with low humidity. However, it's important to clean and maintain the humidifier regularly to prevent the growth of mold and bacteria.

Practice Proper Sinus Care:

Gently blowing your nose one nostril at a time and avoiding forceful nose blowing can prevent further irritation of the nasal passages. Additionally, avoid inserting objects into your nose, such as cotton swabs or fingernails, as it can damage the delicate sinus tissues.

Get Regular Exercise:

Engaging in regular physical exercise is beneficial for overall health, including sinus health. Exercise improves blood circulation and promotes proper drainage of the sinuses. Moderate, intensity exercises, such as brisk walking, swimming, or prenatal yoga, can help reduce the risk of sinusitis.

Manage Stress:

Pregnancy can be a stressful time, and stress can weaken the immune system, making pregnant women more susceptible to infections. Effective stress management techniques, such as meditation, deep breathing exercises, or prenatal yoga, can help reduce stress levels and support a healthy immune system.

Chapter Twenty-Six

The Impact of Pollution on Sinusitis

Sinusitis, an inflammation of the sinuses, can be influenced by various factors, including pollution. Environmental pollution, such as air pollution and indoor pollutants, can have a significant impact on sinus health and contribute to the development or exacerbation of sinusitis. Below we will explore the impact of pollution on sinusitis and discuss the measures that can be taken to minimize its effects.

Air pollution, caused by emissions from vehicles, industrial activities, and the burning of fossil fuels, releases harmful particles and gases into the atmosphere. These pollutants can enter the respiratory system and irritate the nasal passages and sinuses. Fine particulate matter, such as PM2.5, and gaseous pollutants like nitrogen dioxide (NO2) and sulfur dioxide (SO2), can trigger inflammation and worsen symptoms of sinusitis. Long, term exposure to air pollution has been linked to an increased risk of chronic sinusitis.

Indoor pollutants, including volatile organic compounds (VOCs), tobacco smoke, dust mites, mold, and pet dander, can also contribute to sinus inflammation. Poor ventilation and inadequate air filtration systems in homes and workplaces can lead to the accumulation of these pollutants, causing nasal congestion, sinus pressure, and increased susceptibility to sinusitis.

The impact of pollution on sinusitis can be particularly problematic for individuals living in urban areas with high levels of pollution. People exposed to polluted environments, such as heavy traffic areas or industrial zones, may experience more frequent and severe sinusitis symptoms. Additionally, those with pre, existing sinus conditions may find their symptoms worsen in polluted environments.

The inflammatory response triggered by pollution can impair the normal functioning of the sinuses. The nasal mucosa, which lines the sinus cavities, becomes inflamed and swollen, leading to a blockage of the sinus openings. This blockage prevents proper drainage of mucus from the sinuses, creating an ideal environment for the growth of bacteria or viruses and increasing the likelihood of sinusitis.

To minimize the impact of pollution on sinusitis, several preventive measures can be taken:

Reduce Exposure to Outdoor Pollution:

Limit outdoor activities during times of high pollution, such as during rush hour or on days with poor air quality. Check air quality indexes and forecasts to plan outdoor activities when pollution levels are lower. When venturing outdoors, consider wearing a mask specifically designed to filter out pollutants.

Improve Indoor Air Quality:

Ensure proper ventilation in your home by opening windows or using exhaust fans. Use air purifiers or filters to remove pollutants from indoor air. Regularly clean and vacuum your living space to minimize dust and allergens. Avoid smoking and keep your home smoke, free.

Use Nasal Protection:

Consider using nasal filters or nasal irrigation techniques, such as saline nasal sprays or neti pots, to flush out pollutants and keep nasal passages clear. These measures can help reduce the exposure of the sinuses to pollutants and alleviate symptoms of sinusitis.

Maintain Good Hygiene:

Practicing good hygiene, such as frequent handwashing, can minimize the transfer of pollutants from your hands to your nasal passages. Avoid touching your face, especially your nose and eyes, to prevent introducing pollutants into your sinuses.

Strengthen Your Immune System:

A strong immune system can help defend against the harmful effects of pollution on the sinuses. Eat a balanced diet rich in fruits, vegetables, and antioxidants to support immune function. Stay hydrated, exercise regularly, and get adequate sleep to maintain overall health and strengthen your immune system.

Seek Medical Advice:

If you experience persistent or worsening sinusitis symptoms despite preventive measures, consult a healthcare professional. They can provide a proper diagnosis, recommend appropriate treatment options, and offer guidance on managing sinusitis in polluted environments.

Air Pollution and Sinusitis

Sinusitis, a condition characterized by inflammation of the sinuses, can be influenced by various environmental factors, including air pollution. Air pollution, a global issue affecting many cities and industrial areas, can have a significant impact on sinus health and contribute to the development or exacerbation of sinusitis. Below we will explore the relationship between air pollution and sinusitis, discussing the effects of pollutants on sinus health and measures to mitigate their impact.

Air pollution consists of harmful particles and gases released into the atmosphere from various sources, such as industrial activities, vehicle emissions, and the burning of fossil fuels. These pollutants can penetrate the respiratory system and irritate the nasal passages and sinuses, leading to inflammation and other sinusitis symptoms. Fine particulate matter, known as PM2.5, and gaseous pollutants like nitrogen dioxide (NO2) and sulfur dioxide (SO2), are particularly problematic and can worsen sinusitis symptoms.

One of the ways air pollution affects sinus health is by triggering and exacerbating inflammation in the nasal passages and sinuses. When pollutants enter the respiratory system, they can irritate the delicate lining of the sinuses, causing swelling and congestion. This swelling can obstruct the sinus openings and impede the normal flow of mucus, leading to a buildup of mucus and providing an ideal environment for the growth of bacteria or viruses. This, in turn, increases the risk of developing sinusitis.

Long, term exposure to air pollution has been associated with an increased prevalence of chronic sinusitis. Individuals living in areas with high levels of pollution, such as densely populated cities or regions near industrial facilities, may experience more frequent and severe sinusitis symptoms. Furthermore, those with pre, existing sinus conditions may find that their symptoms worsen in polluted environments.

Air pollution can also have a detrimental effect on the immune system, making individuals more susceptible to sinusitis. Prolonged exposure to pollutants can weaken the immune response, reducing the body's ability to fight off infections and increasing the likelihood of sinusitis development.

Additionally, pollutants can interact with allergens and other irritants in the air, exacerbating allergic reactions and sinus inflammation.

To minimize the impact of air pollution on sinusitis, it is important to take proactive measures:

Monitor Air Quality:

Stay informed about the air quality in your area by checking local air quality indexes or using air quality monitoring apps. Plan outdoor activities during times of lower pollution levels, such as early morning or late evening when traffic and industrial activities are reduced.

Limit Outdoor Exposure:

When pollution levels are high, it is advisable to limit outdoor activities, especially in areas with heavy traffic or industrial emissions. Consider using a face mask specifically designed to filter out pollutants when necessary.

Improve Indoor Air Quality:

Create a clean and healthy indoor environment by ensuring proper ventilation and using air purifiers or filters to remove pollutants from the air. Regularly clean and dust your living space to minimize indoor allergens and pollutants. Avoid smoking and keep your home smoke, free.

Promote Respiratory Health:

Maintain good respiratory health by practicing deep breathing exercises, such as diaphragmatic breathing, to strengthen the respiratory muscles and promote proper airflow. Regular exercise can also improve lung function and help the body better cope with the effects of air pollution.

Support Immune Function:

Adopt a healthy lifestyle that includes a balanced diet rich in antioxidants and immune, boosting nutrients. Stay hydrated, get adequate sleep, manage stress levels, and consider taking supplements, if needed, to support immune function and overall health.

Seek Medical Advice:

If you experience persistent or worsening sinusitis symptoms despite taking preventive measures, it is important to seek medical advice. A healthcare professional can provide a proper diagnosis, offer appropriate treatment options.

Indoor Air Quality and Sinus Health

The quality of the air we breathe indoors plays a crucial role in our overall health and well, being, including the health of our sinuses. Poor indoor air quality can contribute to the development and worsening of sinusitis, a condition characterized by inflammation of the sinuses. Below we will explore the impact of indoor air quality on sinus health, discussing common indoor pollutants, their effects on the sinuses, and measures to improve indoor air quality.

Indoor air can be contaminated with various pollutants that can irritate the nasal passages and sinuses, leading to inflammation and sinusitis symptoms. Common indoor pollutants include:

Dust and Allergens:

Dust mites, pet dander, pollen, and mold spores are common allergens that can trigger allergic reactions and sinusitis symptoms. When inhaled, these particles can cause irritation and inflammation in the nasal passages and sinuses.

Volatile Organic Compounds (VOCs):

VOCs are chemicals found in many household products, such as cleaning supplies, paints, varnishes, and air fresheners. Prolonged exposure to VOCs can irritate the respiratory system and contribute to sinusitis symptoms.

Tobacco Smoke:

Exposure to secondhand smoke or smoking itself can have detrimental effects on sinus health. The chemicals in tobacco smoke can irritate the nasal passages, impair the cilia (hair, like structures that help move mucus), and increase the risk of sinus infections.

Household Chemicals:

Cleaning products, pesticides, and other household chemicals can release toxic fumes that can irritate the sinuses and contribute to sinusitis. Proper ventilation and careful use of these products are essential to minimize exposure.

The effects of poor indoor air quality on sinus health can be significant. Individuals with pre, existing sinus conditions may experience more frequent and severe sinusitis symptoms in environments with poor air quality. Additionally, prolonged exposure to indoor pollutants can increase the risk of developing sinusitis or worsen existing sinusitis symptoms.

To improve indoor air quality and promote sinus health, consider the following measures:

Proper Ventilation:

Ensure adequate ventilation in your home to reduce the concentration of indoor pollutants. Open windows and doors whenever possible to allow fresh air to circulate. Use exhaust fans in bathrooms and kitchens to remove moisture and odors.

Regular Cleaning:

Regularly clean your home to reduce dust, allergens, and other particles. Vacuum carpets and upholstery, dust surfaces, and wash bedding frequently. Consider using a vacuum cleaner with a HEPA filter to effectively trap small particles.

Maintain Humidity Levels:

Keep indoor humidity levels between 30% and 50% to discourage the growth of mold and dust mites. Use dehumidifiers in humid environments and consider using a humidifier in dry environments to maintain optimal humidity levels.

Minimize Allergen Exposure:

Take steps to minimize exposure to common allergens. Use dust mite, proof covers for pillows and mattresses, regularly wash bedding in hot water, and keep pets out of bedrooms or designated allergy, free areas.

Choose Low, toxicity Products:

Opt for environmentally friendly and low, toxicity household products. Look for cleaning supplies, paints, and other products labeled as "green" or "low VOC." Avoid using aerosol sprays or products with strong fragrances.

No Smoking Policy:

Implement a strict no, smoking policy in your home to protect your sinuses and overall health. Encourage smokers to smoke outside and create designated smoking areas away from entrances and windows.

Air Purifiers:

Consider using air purifiers with HEPA filters to remove airborne particles and allergens. Place them in commonly used areas, such as bedrooms and living rooms, for maximum effectiveness.

Steps to Reduce Exposure

Steps to Reduce Exposure: Improving Indoor Air Quality for Sinusitis

Sinusitis, the inflammation of the sinuses, can be exacerbated by poor indoor air quality. Indoor pollutants can trigger symptoms and make sinusitis worse. To reduce exposure and promote sinus health, it's important to take proactive steps to improve indoor air quality. Below we will explore various measures to reduce exposure to indoor pollutants and create a healthier environment for individuals with sinusitis.

Identify and Remove Allergens:

One of the first steps in reducing exposure to indoor pollutants is to identify and remove common allergens. Dust mites, pet dander, pollen, and mold spores are common triggers for sinusitis. Regularly clean your home to remove dust and vacuum carpets and furniture. Use allergen, proof covers for mattresses and pillows, and wash bedding in hot water to kill dust mites. If you have pets, bathe them regularly and keep them out of bedrooms.

Ventilate Your Home:

Proper ventilation is crucial for maintaining good indoor air quality. Open windows and doors when weather permits to allow fresh air to circulate. Use exhaust fans in kitchens and bathrooms to remove moisture, odors, and pollutants. Consider installing a whole, house ventilation system to ensure a continuous supply of fresh air.

Control Humidity Levels:

Maintaining appropriate humidity levels can prevent the growth of mold and dust mites, which can trigger sinusitis symptoms. Use dehumidifiers in humid areas of your home, such as basements or bathrooms, to reduce excess moisture. In dry climates, consider using humidifiers to add moisture to the air. Aim for a relative humidity level of 30% to 50%.

Keep a Clean Environment:

Regular cleaning is essential for reducing indoor pollutants. Dust and vacuum your home regularly to remove accumulated allergens. Use a vacuum cleaner equipped with a high, efficiency particulate air (HEPA) filter to trap small particles effectively. Pay attention to commonly overlooked areas, such as curtains, blinds, and upholstery, as they can harbor allergens.

Use Natural Cleaning Products:

Many household cleaning products contain harsh chemicals that can worsen sinusitis symptoms. Opt for natural, eco, friendly cleaning products or make your own using simple ingredients like vinegar, baking soda, and lemon juice. These alternatives are less likely to trigger respiratory irritation and are better for the environment.

Avoid Tobacco Smoke:

Tobacco smoke is a potent irritant that can exacerbate sinusitis symptoms. If you smoke, consider quitting. If you live with a smoker, encourage them to smoke outside or in designated areas away from the home's entrances and windows. This will help minimize exposure to secondhand smoke.

Be Mindful of Chemicals:

Chemicals found in household products, such as air fresheners, paints, and solvents, can release harmful volatile organic compounds (VOCs). These chemicals can irritate the respiratory system and worsen sinusitis symptoms. Opt for low, VOC or VOC, free products, and ensure proper ventilation when using these substances.

Invest in Air Purifiers:

Air purifiers with HEPA filters can help remove airborne allergens and pollutants from your indoor environment. Place them strategically in bedrooms and living areas to ensure maximum effectiveness. Regularly clean and maintain the filters to keep the air purifiers functioning optimally.

Regular HVAC Maintenance:

Heating, ventilation, and air conditioning (HVAC) systems can harbor dust, mold, and other allergens if not properly maintained. Schedule regular HVAC maintenance and change filters as recommended by the manufacturer. Clean air ducts and vents to prevent the circulation of contaminants throughout your home.

Chapter Twenty-Seven

Understanding Your Sinusitis Triggers

Understanding Your Sinusitis Triggers: Identifying and Managing the Factors that Worsen Symptoms

Sinusitis, a condition characterized by inflammation of the sinuses, can be triggered by various factors. By understanding your personal sinusitis triggers, you can take proactive steps to manage and reduce the frequency and severity of symptoms. Below we will explore common triggers of sinusitis and strategies to identify and manage them effectively.

Allergens:

Allergens, such as pollen, dust mites, pet dander, and mold spores, are among the most common triggers of sinusitis. If you suspect allergies are contributing to your symptoms, consider undergoing allergy testing to identify specific allergens. Once you know your triggers, you can take steps to minimize exposure, such as using allergy, proof bedding, regularly cleaning your living space, and avoiding outdoor activities during peak allergen seasons.

Environmental Irritants:

Environmental irritants can worsen sinusitis symptoms or trigger flare, ups. These include strong odors, smoke, chemical fumes, and air pollution. Pay attention to your surroundings and avoid exposure to known irritants. Use fragrance, free products, ensure proper ventilation in your home, and limit your time in heavily polluted areas. If you work in an environment with potential irritants, consider discussing possible accommodations with your employer.

Weather Changes:

Weather changes, particularly shifts in temperature, humidity, and atmospheric pressure, can trigger sinusitis symptoms. Some individuals may experience worsened symptoms during cold weather, while others may be affected by dry or humid conditions. Pay attention to weather forecasts and take appropriate measures, such as wearing a scarf to protect your nose and mouth in cold weather or using a humidifier to add moisture to the air in dry environments.

Certain Foods and Beverages:

While food allergies are not a common trigger for sinusitis, certain foods and beverages can exacerbate symptoms in some individuals. Spicy foods, alcohol, caffeine, and dairy products are among the culprits reported by some sinusitis sufferers. Keep a food diary to identify any patterns between your diet and symptom flare, ups. If you notice a correlation, consider eliminating or reducing the consumption of potential trigger foods.

Nasal Irritants:

Irritation of the nasal passages can worsen sinusitis symptoms. Nasal irritants can include strong perfumes, cleaning products, chlorine from swimming pools, and nasal sprays. Avoid exposure to these irritants as much as possible. Choose mild, fragrance, free personal care products, wear a nose clip while swimming, and use nasal sprays only as directed by your healthcare provider.

Stress and Fatigue:

Stress and fatigue can weaken the immune system and increase susceptibility to infections, including sinusitis. Additionally, stress and fatigue can exacerbate existing sinusitis symptoms. Practice stress management techniques, such as relaxation exercises, meditation, and regular exercise. Prioritize sleep and ensure you are getting adequate rest to support your immune system.

Hormonal Changes:

Hormonal changes, particularly in women, can affect sinusitis symptoms. Fluctuations in hormone levels during menstruation, pregnancy, and menopause have been linked to worsened symptoms. Be mindful of these hormonal changes and track any patterns in symptom severity. Discuss hormone, related concerns with your healthcare provider for appropriate management strategies.

Poor Air Quality:

Indoor and outdoor air quality can impact sinusitis symptoms. Poorly ventilated spaces, exposure to pollutants, and high levels of airborne allergens can worsen symptoms. Take steps to improve indoor air quality, such as using air purifiers, keeping windows closed during high, pollution periods, and avoiding smoke, filled environments.

Identifying Triggers

Identifying Triggers: Understanding and Managing Sinusitis

Sinusitis, also known as sinus inflammation, can be a source of significant discomfort and disruption in daily life. Many factors can contribute to the development and exacerbation of sinusitis symptoms, and identifying these triggers is crucial for effective management. Below we will explore common triggers of sinusitis and discuss strategies for identifying and managing them.

Allergens:

Allergens play a significant role in triggering sinusitis symptoms for many individuals. Common allergens include pollen, dust mites, pet dander, mold spores, and certain foods. Allergy testing can help identify specific allergens that may be causing or worsening sinusitis. Once identified, steps can be taken to minimize exposure to these allergens, such as using air purifiers, regularly cleaning and vacuuming the home, keeping windows closed during high pollen seasons, and avoiding known food triggers.

Environmental Irritants:

Environmental irritants, such as strong odors, smoke, chemical fumes, and air pollution, can trigger sinusitis symptoms. Being mindful of your surroundings and avoiding exposure to known irritants is crucial. Ensure proper ventilation in your living spaces, use fragrance, free and hypoallergenic products, and limit your time in heavily polluted areas. If you work in an environment with potential irritants, consider wearing a mask or discussing possible accommodations with your employer.

Weather Changes:

Weather changes, particularly shifts in temperature, humidity, and atmospheric pressure, can impact sinusitis symptoms. Many individuals experience worsened symptoms during cold weather, while others may be affected by dry or humid conditions. Paying attention to weather forecasts can help you anticipate and prepare for potential symptom flare, ups. Protective measures, such as wearing a scarf to cover your nose and mouth in cold weather or using a humidifier to add moisture to the air in dry environments, can be helpful in managing symptoms.

Nasal Irritants:

Irritation of the nasal passages can contribute to sinusitis symptoms. Nasal irritants can include strong perfumes, cleaning products, airborne particles, and nasal sprays. Avoiding exposure to these irritants is important for managing sinusitis. Opt for mild, fragrance, free personal care products, use gentle cleaning agents, and be cautious with nasal sprays. Consult with a healthcare professional before using nasal sprays and follow the recommended guidelines.

Stress and Fatigue:

Stress and fatigue have been known to worsen sinusitis symptoms. When we are stressed or fatigued, our immune system may become compromised, making us more susceptible to infections and inflammation. Engaging in stress management techniques, such as regular exercise, meditation, deep breathing exercises, and adequate rest, can help reduce the impact of stress and fatigue on sinusitis symptoms.

Dietary Factors:

Dietary choices can influence sinusitis symptoms for some individuals. Certain foods and beverages, such as spicy foods, alcohol, caffeine, and dairy products, have been reported to trigger or worsen sinusitis symptoms in some people. Keeping a food diary can help identify any patterns between your diet and symptom flare, ups. If you notice a correlation, consider reducing or eliminating these potential trigger foods from your diet and exploring alternative options.

Hormonal Changes:

Hormonal changes, particularly in women, can affect sinusitis symptoms. Fluctuations in hormone levels during menstrual cycles, pregnancy, and menopause can contribute to increased sinusitis symptoms in some individuals. Being mindful of these hormonal changes and tracking any patterns in symptom severity can help with management. Consulting with a healthcare professional can provide guidance on managing sinusitis symptoms related to hormonal changes.

Sinus Infections:

Sinus infections, whether caused by bacteria or viruses, can trigger or exacerbate sinusitis symptoms.

Managing Trigger Exposure

Managing Trigger Exposure: Minimizing Sinusitis Symptoms

Sinusitis can be a chronic condition that significantly affects daily life. One key aspect of effectively managing sinusitis is to minimize exposure to triggers that can worsen symptoms or lead to sinusitis flare, ups. Identifying and addressing these triggers is crucial for individuals seeking relief. Below we will explore various strategies for managing trigger exposure and reducing the impact of sinusitis on overall well, being.

Allergen Management:

Allergens, such as pollen, dust mites, pet dander, mold spores, and certain foods, can trigger or exacerbate sinusitis symptoms in individuals with allergies. Taking steps to manage allergens is essential. This may include:

Regularly cleaning and vacuuming your home to remove dust and allergens.

Using allergen, proof bedding and pillow covers to minimize exposure to dust mites.

Keeping windows closed during high pollen seasons and using air purifiers to improve indoor air quality.

Washing hands and clothes after outdoor activities to remove potential allergens.

Avoiding known food triggers and working with a healthcare professional to develop a suitable diet plan.

Environmental Control:

Controlling the environment can significantly reduce exposure to irritants and pollutants that can trigger sinusitis symptoms. Consider the following strategies:

Keeping indoor air clean by using air purifiers, ensuring proper ventilation, and avoiding smoking or exposure to secondhand smoke.

Using hypoallergenic cleaning products and minimizing the use of strong chemicals or fragrances.

Taking precautions when exposed to potential irritants such as paint fumes, household cleaners, or strong perfumes.

Paying attention to air quality alerts and avoiding outdoor activities on days with high pollution levels.

Nasal Irrigation:

Nasal irrigation, using a saline solution, can help remove allergens, irritants, and mucus from the nasal passages, providing relief from sinusitis symptoms. Consider using a neti pot or a nasal saline rinse kit to flush the nasal passages gently. However, it is important to use distilled or sterile water and follow proper hygiene practices to prevent any risk of infection.

Proper Hydration:

Staying adequately hydrated is essential for maintaining healthy sinus passages. Drinking enough water can help thin mucus and promote proper drainage, reducing the risk of sinus congestion and infection. Aim to drink plenty of fluids throughout the day, and consider using a humidifier in dry environments to add moisture to the air.

Stress Management:

Stress can weaken the immune system and contribute to increased inflammation and sinusitis symptoms. Incorporating stress management techniques into daily life can help reduce the impact of stress on sinus health. Consider activities such as yoga, meditation, deep breathing exercises, regular exercise, and engaging in hobbies or activities that promote relaxation.

Regular Exercise:

Engaging in regular physical exercise has numerous benefits for overall health, including sinus health. Exercise helps improve blood circulation, boost immune function, and reduce inflammation. However, it is important to be mindful of the environmental conditions while exercising, such as pollution or extreme weather, that can potentially worsen sinusitis symptoms.

Proper Respiratory Hygiene:

Practicing good respiratory hygiene can help minimize the spread of viruses and bacteria that can lead to sinus infections. This includes:

Covering your mouth and nose with a tissue or your elbow when coughing or sneezing.

Washing your hands frequently with soap and water for at least 20 seconds.

Avoiding touching your face, especially your nose and mouth, to reduce the risk of introducing pathogens into the sinuses.

Regular Medical Follow, up:

Regular medical follow, up is essential for individuals with chronic sinusitis. Working with a healthcare professional ensures proper diagnosis, management, and monitoring of sinusitis symptoms.

Personalized Sinusitis Management

Personalized Sinusitis Management: Tailoring Treatment for Effective Relief

Sinusitis is a condition that affects millions of individuals worldwide, causing significant discomfort and impairing quality of life. While general treatment approaches exist, it is important to recognize that each person's experience with sinusitis can be unique. Personalized sinusitis management involves tailoring treatment strategies to address individual needs, triggers, and symptoms. Below we will explore the concept of personalized sinusitis management and discuss various aspects that contribute to effective relief.

Comprehensive Medical Evaluation:

Personalized sinusitis management begins with a comprehensive medical evaluation. This evaluation may include a detailed medical history, physical examination, and diagnostic tests such as imaging studies or nasal endoscopy. These assessments help identify the underlying cause of sinusitis and any specific factors contributing to the symptoms.

Identifying Triggers:

Understanding the triggers that worsen sinusitis symptoms is crucial for personalized management. Triggers can vary among individuals and may include allergens, irritants, weather changes, infections, or underlying health conditions. By identifying and addressing these triggers, individuals can take proactive steps to minimize exposure and reduce symptom severity.

Allergy Testing:

Allergy testing plays a vital role in personalized sinusitis management, especially for individuals with chronic sinusitis. Allergies can contribute to sinus inflammation and exacerbate symptoms. Allergy testing can identify specific allergens that trigger sinusitis and guide targeted treatment approaches such as allergen avoidance, immunotherapy, or medication options.

Medication Management:

Medication management is a key component of personalized sinusitis treatment. Depending on the severity and underlying cause of sinusitis, healthcare professionals may prescribe various medications such as:

Nasal corticosteroids: These medications reduce inflammation in the nasal passages and can provide significant relief for sinusitis symptoms.

Decongestants: Oral or nasal decongestants help relieve nasal congestion, but they should be used with caution and only for short durations to avoid rebound congestion.

Antibiotics: If a bacterial infection is suspected or diagnosed, antibiotics may be prescribed to treat the infection.

Antihistamines: Antihistamines are useful for managing allergic rhinitis symptoms that contribute to sinusitis.

Saline nasal sprays or rinses: These help to irrigate the nasal passages, reduce congestion, and promote sinus drainage.

The choice of medications and their dosage should be personalized based on the individual's specific condition and response to treatment.

Functional Endoscopic Sinus Surgery (FESS):

In cases of chronic or recurrent sinusitis that does not respond well to medication, functional endoscopic sinus surgery (FESS) may be considered. FESS is a minimally invasive surgical procedure that aims to improve sinus drainage and reduce inflammation. It involves the use of an endoscope to remove obstructive tissues or to open blocked sinuses, allowing better airflow and drainage. FESS is typically performed by an ear, nose, and throat (ENT) specialist and is tailored to each individual's unique sinus anatomy and specific needs.

Lifestyle Modifications:

Lifestyle modifications play a crucial role in personalized sinusitis management. Adopting healthy habits and making positive changes can contribute to overall sinus health. Some lifestyle modifications to consider include:

Maintaining proper hydration: Drinking plenty of water helps thin mucus and promote effective sinus drainage.

Practicing good nasal hygiene: Regularly cleaning the nasal passages with saline nasal sprays or rinses can help reduce mucus build, up and keep the sinuses clear.

Avoiding smoking and secondhand smoke: Smoking can irritate the respiratory system and worsen sinusitis symptoms.

Chapter Twenty-Eight

Sinusitis Myths and Misconceptions

Sinusitis Myths and Misconceptions: Separating Fact from Fiction

Sinusitis is a common condition that affects many individuals worldwide. Unfortunately, it is also surrounded by various myths and misconceptions that can lead to misunderstandings about the condition and its treatment. Below we will we aim to debunk some of the most prevalent sinusitis myths and provide factual information to enhance understanding and promote effective management.

Myth 1: Sinusitis is just a bad cold.

Fact: While sinusitis can develop as a result of a cold or respiratory infection, it is not merely a severe cold. Sinusitis occurs when the sinuses, which are air, filled cavities in the skull, become inflamed and infected. It can be acute (lasting less than four weeks) or chronic (lasting more than 12 weeks). Sinusitis symptoms often include facial pain or pressure, nasal congestion, headache, and thick nasal discharge.

Myth 2: Antibiotics are always necessary for treating sinusitis.

Fact: Antibiotics are not always required for treating sinusitis. In fact, most cases of acute sinusitis are caused by viruses and do not respond to antibiotics. Antibiotics should be prescribed only when bacterial infection is confirmed or suspected. Overuse or misuse of antibiotics can contribute to antibiotic resistance and other potential side effects.

Myth 3: Sinusitis is contagious.

Fact: Sinusitis itself is not contagious. However, the infections that sometimes lead to sinusitis, such as the common cold or flu, can be contagious. It is important to practice good hygiene, such as frequent handwashing, to reduce the risk of spreading respiratory infections.

Myth 4: Sinusitis always requires surgery.

Fact: Surgery is not the first, line treatment for sinusitis. Most cases of sinusitis can be effectively managed with non, surgical approaches, including medication, saline nasal irrigation, and lifestyle modifications. Surgery, such as functional endoscopic sinus surgery (FESS), is typically considered only for chronic or recurrent sinusitis that does not respond well to conservative treatments.

Myth 5: Sinusitis is only caused by allergies.

Fact: While allergies can contribute to sinusitis, they are not the only cause. Sinusitis can be triggered by various factors, including viral or bacterial infections, structural abnormalities in the sinuses, nasal polyps, or immune system disorders. Identifying and addressing the underlying cause of sinusitis is crucial for effective management.

Myth 6: Sinusitis only affects adults.

Fact: Sinusitis can affect individuals of all ages, including children. In fact, chronic sinusitis is often seen in children with underlying conditions such as allergies or immune system disorders. It is important to recognize and seek appropriate treatment for sinusitis in children to alleviate their symptoms and prevent complications.

Myth 7: Nasal congestion means you have sinusitis.

Fact: Nasal congestion can be a symptom of sinusitis, but it can also occur due to other factors such as allergies, the common cold, or nasal polyps. A thorough medical evaluation is necessary to determine the cause of nasal congestion and related symptoms.

Myth 8: Sinusitis can be cured with natural remedies alone.

Fact: While natural remedies such as saline nasal irrigation, steam inhalation, or herbal supplements may provide temporary relief, they are not a cure, all for sinusitis. In cases of chronic or severe sinusitis, medical intervention and appropriate medications may be necessary to effectively manage the condition.

Myth 9: Sinusitis always requires a long recovery period.

Fact: The recovery period for sinusitis varies depending on the severity and underlying cause. Acute sinusitis often resolves within a few weeks with appropriate treatment.

Common Sinusitis Myths

Common Sinusitis Myths: Debunking Misconceptions for Better Understanding

Sinusitis is a widespread condition that affects millions of people worldwide. Unfortunately, there are many myths and misconceptions surrounding this common ailment. These misunderstandings can lead to ineffective management and unnecessary worry. Below we will debunk some of the most prevalent sinusitis myths and provide factual information to promote a better understanding of the condition.

Myth 1: Sinusitis is just a severe headache.

Fact: While headaches can be a symptom of sinusitis, it is not limited to head pain. Sinusitis is the inflammation of the sinuses, which are air, filled cavities in the skull. Common symptoms include facial pain or pressure, nasal congestion, thick nasal discharge, and decreased sense of smell. Headaches associated with sinusitis are often localized in the forehead, cheeks, or between the eyes.

Myth 2: Sinusitis is always caused by allergies.

Fact: While allergies can trigger sinusitis in some individuals, it is not the sole cause. Sinusitis can also result from viral or bacterial infections, nasal polyps, deviated septum, or structural abnormalities in the sinuses. Identifying the underlying cause is essential for proper treatment and management of sinusitis.

Myth 3: Antibiotics are always necessary for treating sinusitis.

Fact: Antibiotics are not always required for sinusitis treatment. Most cases of acute sinusitis are caused by viruses and do not respond to antibiotics. In such cases, the focus should be on managing symptoms with over, the, counter pain relievers, nasal saline rinses, and steam inhalation. Antibiotics are only recommended if bacterial infection is suspected or confirmed.

Myth 4: Sinusitis is contagious.

Fact: Sinusitis itself is not contagious. However, the viruses or bacteria that can cause sinusitis can be transmitted from person to person. Respiratory infections like the common cold or flu, which can lead to sinusitis, are contagious. Practicing good hand hygiene and avoiding close contact with infected individuals can help reduce the risk of contracting respiratory infections.

Myth 5: Surgery is the only solution for chronic sinusitis.

Fact: Surgery is not the first, line treatment for chronic sinusitis. In most cases, chronic sinusitis can be effectively managed with medical therapies, including nasal corticosteroids, saline irrigation, and allergy treatments. Surgery, such as functional endoscopic sinus surgery (FESS), is considered when conservative measures fail or when there are structural abnormalities that require correction.

Myth 6: Sinusitis is a lifelong condition.

Fact: While some individuals may experience recurrent or chronic sinusitis, it is not necessarily a lifelong condition. With proper management, many people can effectively control their symptoms and reduce the frequency and severity of sinusitis episodes. Identifying triggers, following a sinus, friendly lifestyle, and seeking appropriate medical care are key to managing sinusitis effectively.

Myth 7: Sinusitis is always accompanied by yellow or green nasal discharge.

Fact: The color of nasal discharge does not determine the presence or absence of sinusitis. While yellow or green discharge can indicate an infection, clear or white discharge can also be present in sinusitis. The consistency of the discharge, along with other symptoms like facial pain, pressure, or congestion, should be considered when evaluating sinusitis.

Myth 8: Sinusitis only affects adults.

Fact: Sinusitis can affect individuals of all ages, including children. Children may experience acute or chronic sinusitis due to respiratory infections, allergies, or anatomical factors. It is essential to recognize and seek appropriate medical care for children with sinusitis to alleviate their symptoms and prevent complications.

The Truth About Sinusitis

The Truth About Sinusitis: Dispelling Myths and Providing Facts for a Better Understanding

Sinusitis is a condition that affects millions of people worldwide, causing discomfort and impacting daily life. Unfortunately, there are numerous myths and misconceptions surrounding sinusitis that can lead to confusion and misinformation. Below we will separate fact from fiction and provide a clear understanding of sinusitis, its causes, symptoms, and treatments.

Myth 1: Sinusitis is just a common cold.

Fact: While sinusitis can develop as a result of a cold or flu, it is not the same as a common cold. Sinusitis refers to the inflammation of the sinuses, which are air, filled cavities located in the skull. It can be acute or chronic and may persist long after the initial respiratory infection has resolved.

Myth 2: Sinusitis is always caused by allergies.

Fact: While allergies can contribute to sinusitis, it is not the sole cause. Sinusitis can also be triggered by bacterial or viral infections, structural abnormalities in the nasal passages, nasal polyps, or a weakened immune system. It is essential to identify the underlying cause to determine the most appropriate treatment approach.

Myth 3: Antibiotics are always necessary for treating sinusitis.

Fact: Antibiotics are not always required for sinusitis treatment. In fact, most cases of acute sinusitis are caused by viral infections, which do not respond to antibiotics. Antibiotics should only be prescribed when there is evidence of a bacterial infection. Proper diagnosis and evaluation by a healthcare professional are crucial in determining the need for antibiotics.

Myth 4: Sinusitis is a chronic condition that cannot be cured.

Fact: While chronic sinusitis may require ongoing management, it can be effectively controlled and its symptoms minimized. Treatment options, such as nasal saline rinses, nasal corticosteroids, decongestants, and allergy medications, can help alleviate symptoms and improve quality of life. In some cases, surgery may be necessary to correct underlying structural issues.

Myth 5: Sinusitis only affects the nasal passages.

Fact: Sinusitis affects not only the nasal passages but also the surrounding sinuses. The sinuses are air, filled cavities connected to the nasal passages. Inflammation and congestion can block the sinus openings, leading to pain, pressure, and other symptoms. Sinusitis can also cause referred pain, such as headaches, toothaches, or facial pain.

Myth 6: Sinusitis is contagious.

Fact: Sinusitis itself is not contagious. However, the underlying conditions that contribute to sinusitis, such as colds, flu, or allergies, can be contagious. It is important to practice good hygiene, such as handwashing and avoiding close contact with individuals who have respiratory infections, to reduce the risk of contracting these conditions.

Myth 7: Sinusitis can only be treated with medication.

Fact: While medication is often a part of sinusitis treatment, it is not the sole approach. Home remedies and lifestyle changes can play a significant role in managing sinusitis. Nasal saline rinses, steam inhalation, warm compresses, adequate hydration, and avoiding triggers such as allergens or irritants can help alleviate symptoms and promote healing.

Myth 8: Surgery is always required for chronic sinusitis.

Fact: Surgery is typically reserved for cases of chronic sinusitis that do not respond to conservative treatments. It is not the first, line treatment option. Non, surgical approaches, such as nasal corticosteroids, nasal saline rinses, and allergy management, are usually recommended as initial treatment strategies. Surgery may be considered if there are structural abnormalities or recurrent infections.

Dispelling Fear and Misinformation

Dispelling Fear and Misinformation: Clearing the Air on Sinusitis

Sinusitis is a common condition that affects millions of people worldwide. Unfortunately, there are several myths and misconceptions surrounding sinusitis that can lead to fear, confusion, and unnecessary anxiety. Below we will debunk these myths and provide factual information to help individuals gain a better understanding of sinusitis.

Myth 1: Sinusitis is a life, threatening condition.

Fact: While sinusitis can cause discomfort and affect daily life, it is not typically a life, threatening condition. Most cases of sinusitis are acute and can be effectively managed with proper treatment and self, care measures. However, chronic sinusitis may require ongoing management to alleviate symptoms and improve quality of life.

Myth 2: Sinusitis always requires antibiotics.

Fact: Antibiotics are not always necessary for treating sinusitis. In fact, the majority of sinusitis cases are caused by viral infections, which do not respond to antibiotics. Antibiotics are only recommended when there is evidence of a bacterial infection or when symptoms persist despite conservative treatments. It is important to consult with a healthcare professional to determine the most appropriate treatment approach.

Myth 3: Sinusitis is contagious.

Fact: Sinusitis itself is not contagious. However, the underlying conditions that contribute to sinusitis, such as colds or flu, can be contagious. Sinusitis is often preceded by a viral infection, which can spread from person to person. Practicing good hygiene, such as frequent handwashing, can help reduce the risk of contracting or spreading respiratory infections.

Myth 4: Sinusitis is only caused by allergies.

Fact: While allergies can contribute to sinusitis, it is not the sole cause. Sinusitis can also be triggered by bacterial or viral infections, structural abnormalities in the nasal passages, nasal polyps, or a weakened immune system. It is important to identify the underlying cause of sinusitis to determine the most appropriate treatment plan.

Myth 5: Sinusitis is a result of poor hygiene.

Fact: Sinusitis is not solely caused by poor hygiene. While maintaining good hygiene, such as regular handwashing and keeping the nasal passages clean, can help reduce the risk of respiratory infections, it is not the sole determinant of sinusitis. Other factors, such as allergies, anatomical abnormalities, or a compromised immune system, can also contribute to the development of sinusitis.

Myth 6: Sinusitis always requires surgery.

Fact: Surgery is not the first, line treatment for sinusitis. In most cases, sinusitis can be effectively managed with conservative treatments such as nasal saline rinses, nasal corticosteroids, decongestants, and pain relievers. Surgery is typically reserved for individuals with chronic sinusitis who do not respond to conservative treatments or have structural abnormalities that require correction.

Myth 7: Sinusitis can be cured with over, the, counter medications.

Fact: Over, the, counter medications can provide temporary relief of symptoms, but they cannot cure sinusitis. Sinusitis treatment involves a comprehensive approach that may include prescription medications, lifestyle modifications, and self, care measures. It is important to consult with a healthcare professional for an accurate diagnosis and appropriate treatment plan.

Myth 8: Sinusitis is a normal part of aging.

Fact: While the risk of developing sinusitis may increase with age, it is not a normal part of the aging process. Sinusitis can affect individuals of all ages, and its development is influenced by various factors such as allergies, infections, and structural abnormalities. It is important to address the underlying causes and manage symptoms effectively, regardless of age.

Chapter Twenty-Nine

Your Sinusitis Action Plan

Your Sinusitis Action Plan: Taking Control of Sinusitis

Living with sinusitis can be challenging, but with a well, defined action plan, you can take control of your symptoms and improve your quality of life. Below we will discuss the key components of a comprehensive sinusitis action plan that includes prevention strategies, symptom management, and proactive measures to minimize the impact of sinusitis on your daily life.

Understanding Sinusitis

To develop an effective action plan, it is important to have a clear understanding of sinusitis. Sinusitis is an inflammation of the sinuses, which are air, filled cavities located in the facial bones around the nose and eyes. It can be caused by various factors, including allergies, infections, and anatomical abnormalities. The symptoms of sinusitis often include facial pain, congestion, nasal discharge, and headaches.

Prevention Strategies

Preventing sinusitis starts with understanding and avoiding your personal triggers. Common triggers include allergens, irritants, and respiratory infections. To prevent sinusitis:

a. Identify and manage your allergies: If you have allergies, work with a healthcare professional to develop an allergy management plan that includes allergen avoidance, medications, and immunotherapy if necessary.

b. Maintain good nasal hygiene: Rinse your nasal passages with saline solution regularly to flush out irritants and promote sinus health.

c. Practice good hand hygiene: Wash your hands frequently, especially during the cold and flu seasons, to reduce the risk of respiratory infections.

d. Avoid environmental irritants: Minimize your exposure to cigarette smoke, air pollution, and other irritants that can trigger sinusitis symptoms.

Symptom Management

When sinusitis symptoms flare up, it is important to have strategies in place to manage them effectively. Consider the following approaches:

a. Nasal irrigation: Use a saline nasal rinse or spray to keep your nasal passages moist and clear of mucus.

b. Steam inhalation: Inhaling steam from a bowl of hot water or using a facial steamer can help alleviate congestion and promote sinus drainage.

c. Over, the, counter medications: Non, prescription pain relievers, decongestants, and nasal sprays may provide temporary relief of symptoms. However, use them judiciously and follow the instructions carefully.

d. Prescription medications: If your symptoms are severe or persistent, consult a healthcare professional who may prescribe nasal corticosteroids, antibiotics (if a bacterial infection is present), or other medications to manage your sinusitis.

Lifestyle Modifications

Certain lifestyle habits can exacerbate sinusitis symptoms or increase your susceptibility to sinusitis. Consider making the following changes to support sinus health:

a. Stay hydrated: Drink plenty of fluids to keep your nasal passages hydrated and promote proper mucus flow.

b. Maintain a healthy diet: Eat a balanced diet rich in fruits, vegetables, and whole grains to support your immune system and overall health.

c. Avoid triggers: Identify and avoid specific triggers that worsen your sinusitis symptoms. This may include certain foods, environmental allergens, or lifestyle factors such as smoking.

d. Manage stress: Stress can weaken the immune system and exacerbate sinusitis symptoms. Incorporate stress management techniques such as exercise, meditation, and relaxation techniques into your daily routine.

Proactive Measures

In addition to prevention, symptom management, and lifestyle modifications, proactive measures can help minimize the impact of sinusitis on your daily life:

a. Regular check, ups: Maintain regular visits with your healthcare professional to monitor your sinus health, discuss any changes in symptoms, and adjust your treatment plan if necessary.

b. Communication with your healthcare team: Keep an open line of communication with your healthcare professional. Share your concerns, ask questions, and actively participate in your treatment plan.

Developing a Management Plan

Developing a Management Plan: Taking Charge of Your Sinusitis

Living with sinusitis can be challenging, but with a well, developed management plan, you can effectively control your symptoms and improve your quality of life. Below we will discuss the key components of a comprehensive sinusitis management plan that includes prevention strategies, symptom management techniques, and proactive measures to minimize the impact of sinusitis on your daily life.

Understanding Sinusitis

Before developing a management plan, it is important to have a clear understanding of sinusitis. Sinusitis is an inflammation of the sinuses, which are hollow spaces in the facial bones surrounding the nasal cavity. It can be caused by various factors such as allergies, infections, or structural abnormalities. Common symptoms of sinusitis include facial pain, nasal congestion, post, nasal drip, and headaches.

Prevention Strategies

Prevention is an essential part of managing sinusitis. By identifying and avoiding triggers, you can significantly reduce the frequency and severity of sinusitis episodes. Consider the following prevention strategies:

Allergen Management: If allergies are a trigger for your sinusitis, work with an allergist to identify specific allergens and develop an appropriate management plan. This may include allergen avoidance, medication, or immunotherapy.

Nasal Irrigation: Regularly rinsing your nasal passages with a saline solution can help remove irritants, reduce inflammation, and promote sinus health.

Environmental Control: Minimize your exposure to environmental irritants such as cigarette smoke, air pollution, and strong odors, as they can aggravate sinusitis symptoms.

Hand Hygiene: Practicing good hand hygiene, especially during the cold and flu seasons, can reduce the risk of respiratory infections that can trigger sinusitis.

Symptom Management

When sinusitis symptoms arise, it is important to have effective strategies to alleviate discomfort and manage symptoms. Consider the following approaches:

Nasal Saline Sprays: Using over, the, counter saline sprays or nasal rinses can help moisturize and clear your nasal passages, reducing congestion and facilitating mucus drainage.

Warm Compresses: Applying warm compresses to your face can help relieve facial pain and pressure associated with sinusitis.

Steam Inhalation: Inhaling steam from a bowl of hot water or using a steam inhaler can help soothe irritated nasal passages, loosen mucus, and improve breathing.

Medications: Over, the, counter pain relievers, decongestants, and nasal corticosteroids may provide temporary relief from sinusitis symptoms. However, it is important to use them as directed and consult with a healthcare professional if symptoms persist.

Proactive Measures

In addition to prevention and symptom management, proactive measures can help you stay ahead of sinusitis and minimize its impact on your daily life:

Regular Follow, ups: Schedule regular check, ups with your healthcare provider to monitor your sinus health, discuss any changes in symptoms, and adjust your treatment plan if necessary.

Communication with Healthcare Providers: Maintain open and ongoing communication with your healthcare team. Share your concerns, ask questions, and actively participate in the development and adjustment of your management plan.

Lifestyle Modifications: Certain lifestyle changes can support sinus health and reduce the frequency of sinusitis episodes. These may include:

a. Quitting smoking: Smoking irritates the nasal passages and can worsen sinusitis symptoms. Quitting smoking can improve sinus health and overall well, being.

b. Healthy Diet and Hydration: Eating a well, balanced diet rich in fruits, vegetables, and whole grains can support immune function and reduce inflammation. Staying hydrated by drinking plenty of fluids can help maintain adequate moisture in your nasal passages.

When to Seek Medical Help

Knowing When to Seek Medical Help: Managing Sinusitis Effectively

Sinusitis is a common condition that affects millions of people worldwide. While many cases of sinusitis can be managed at home with self, care measures, there are times when medical intervention is necessary. Below we will explore the signs and symptoms that indicate it is time to seek medical help for sinusitis. It is important to remember that everyone's condition is unique, and consulting a healthcare professional is the best way to determine the appropriate course of action.

Understanding Sinusitis

Sinusitis is an inflammation of the sinuses, which are air, filled spaces located in the facial bones around the nose and eyes. It can be caused by various factors, including infections, allergies, and structural abnormalities. Common symptoms of sinusitis include facial pain, nasal congestion, thick nasal discharge, post, nasal drip, and pressure around the eyes or forehead.

Self, Care Measures

In many cases, mild to moderate sinusitis can be managed effectively with self, care measures. These include:

Nasal Irrigation: Using a saline solution or nasal rinse to flush out the nasal passages can help relieve congestion and promote sinus drainage.

Steam Inhalation: Inhaling steam from a bowl of hot water or using a steam inhaler can help soothe the nasal passages and alleviate symptoms.

Warm Compresses: Applying warm compresses to the face can help reduce facial pain and pressure.

Hydration: Staying hydrated by drinking plenty of fluids can help thin the mucus and promote better sinus drainage.

Rest and Sleep: Getting adequate rest and sleep allows the body to heal and recover, boosting the immune system's ability to fight off infections.

When to Seek Medical Help

While self, care measures can provide relief for many individuals, there are situations when it is crucial to seek medical help. Here are some indications that medical intervention is necessary:

Severe or Prolonged Symptoms: If your sinusitis symptoms are severe, persist for more than 10 days, or worsen over time despite self, care measures, it is advisable to consult a healthcare professional. Severe symptoms may include severe facial pain, high fever, or worsening headache.

Recurrent Sinusitis: If you experience recurrent sinusitis episodes, with symptoms recurring multiple times within a year, medical attention is recommended. This may indicate an underlying issue that needs further evaluation and treatment.

Suspected Complications: If you develop complications related to sinusitis, such as the spread of infection to the eye, brain, or surrounding tissues, it is crucial to seek immediate medical help. Symptoms of complications may include severe headache, vision changes, double vision, swelling around the eyes, or high fever.

Worsening Allergy Symptoms: If your sinusitis is caused by allergies and your allergy symptoms are worsening, despite taking allergy medications, it is important to consult with an allergist or an ENT specialist. They can help identify triggers, provide appropriate treatment options, and manage your condition effectively.

Impact on Daily Life: If sinusitis significantly impacts your daily life, interfering with work, school, or other activities, it is essential to seek medical help. Chronic sinusitis can affect your overall well, being, productivity, and quality of life, and a healthcare professional can offer tailored treatment options to alleviate your symptoms.

Medical Interventions

When you seek medical help for sinusitis, your healthcare provider will assess your symptoms, medical history, and perform a physical examination. They may recommend the following interventions:

Antibiotics: If your sinusitis is caused by a bacterial infection or if there is a secondary bacterial infection, your healthcare provider may prescribe antibiotics to help fight the infection.

Staying Proactive in Your Sinus Health

Staying Proactive in Your Sinus Health: Taking Control of Sinusitis

Sinusitis is a common condition that can cause significant discomfort and affect your overall quality of life. While there are various factors that contribute to sinusitis, it is important to take a proactive approach to manage and prevent its recurrence. Below we will explore practical strategies and lifestyle adjustments that can help you stay proactive in maintaining your sinus health.

Understanding Sinusitis

Sinusitis, also known as a sinus infection, is the inflammation of the sinuses, which are hollow spaces located in the facial bones around the nose and eyes. It can be caused by infections, allergies, structural abnormalities, or other factors. Common symptoms of sinusitis include facial pain, nasal congestion, headache, post, nasal drip, and a reduced sense of smell.

Taking Control: Staying Proactive

Maintain Good Nasal Hygiene

Proper nasal hygiene is crucial in preventing and managing sinusitis. Here are some key practices to incorporate into your daily routine:

a. Nasal Irrigation: Regularly rinsing your nasal passages with a saline solution can help remove irritants, allergens, and mucus, promoting sinus health. Use a neti pot, nasal spray, or squeeze bottle designed for nasal irrigation.

b. Keep Your Sinuses Moist: Dry sinuses can lead to irritation and inflammation. Use a humidifier to add moisture to the air, especially in dry environments or during winter months.

c. Avoid Irritants: Minimize exposure to irritants such as smoke, strong chemical odors, and airborne pollutants, as they can aggravate your sinuses.

Manage Allergies

Allergies can significantly contribute to sinusitis. If you have allergies, take proactive steps to manage them:

a. Identify Triggers: Work with an allergist to identify your specific allergens. This may involve undergoing allergy testing, such as skin prick tests or blood tests.

b. Allergy Medications: Follow your healthcare provider's recommendations for allergy medications, such as antihistamines or nasal corticosteroids, to alleviate symptoms and reduce inflammation.

c. Environmental Control: Take measures to minimize exposure to allergens, such as keeping windows closed during high pollen seasons, using dust mite covers on bedding, and regularly cleaning your living spaces.

Boost Your Immune System

A strong immune system is essential in preventing and fighting off infections that can lead to sinusitis. Here are some ways to support your immune health:

a. Balanced Diet: Consume a well, rounded diet rich in fruits, vegetables, whole grains, and lean proteins to provide your body with the necessary nutrients for optimal immune function.

b. Regular Exercise: Engage in regular physical activity to boost your overall immune system and promote healthy blood circulation.

c. Sufficient Rest and Sleep: Prioritize quality sleep to allow your body to recover and maintain a strong immune system.

Practice Good Sinus Care During Travel

Traveling can expose you to different environments and potential triggers for sinusitis. Follow these tips to stay proactive during your travels:

a. Stay Hydrated: Drink plenty of fluids, especially during air travel, to prevent dehydration and maintain moist sinus passages.

b. Use Nasal Sprays: Consider using nasal saline sprays or nasal moisturizing gels during flights to keep your sinuses moisturized and reduce the risk of congestion.

c. Be Mindful of Environmental Triggers: Avoid exposure to known triggers, such as smoke, dust, and strong odors, that can irritate your sinuses.

* 9 7 8 1 7 7 6 8 4 6 9 2 4 *
SD - #0022 - 140926 - C0 - 229/152/17 - PB - 9781776846924 - Matt Lamination